Doing
a Literature
Review in
Nursing, Health
and Social Care

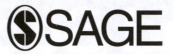
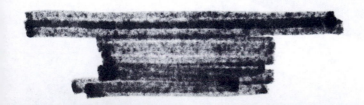

Doing a Literature Review in Nursing, Health and Social Care

Michael Coughlan,
Patricia Cronin and
Frances Ryan

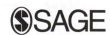

Los Angeles | London | New Delhi
Singapore | Washington DC

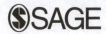

Los Angeles | London | New Delhi
Singapore | Washington DC

SAGE Publications Ltd
1 Oliver's Yard
55 City Road
London EC1Y 1SP

SAGE Publications Inc.
2455 Teller Road
Thousand Oaks, California 91320

SAGE Publications India Pvt Ltd
B 1/I 1 Mohan Cooperative Industrial Area
Mathura Road
New Delhi 110 044

SAGE Publications Asia-Pacific Pte Ltd
3 Church Street
#10-04 Samsung Hub
Singapore 049483

Editor: Alex Clabburn
Assistant editor: Emma Milman
Production editor: Katie Forsythe
Copyeditor: William Baginsky
Proofreader: Neil Dowden
Indexer: Silvia Benvenuto
Marketing manager: Tamara Navaratnam
Cover design: Wendy Scott
Typeset by: C&M Digitals (P) Ltd, Chennai, India
Printed and bound by Bell & Bain Ltd, Glasgow

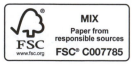

MIX
Paper from
responsible sources
FSC® C007785
www.fsc.org

Library of Congress Control Number: 2012948271

British Library Cataloguing in Publication data

A catalogue record for this book is available from the British Library

ISBN 978-1-4462-4960-4
ISBN 978-1-4462-4961-1 (pbk)

Contents

Figures and Tables   vii

About the Authors   ix

1 What is a Literature Review?   1

2 Types of Literature Review   8

3 Systematic Review   32

4 Selecting a Review Topic and Searching the Literature   48

5 Reading and Organising the Literature   62

6 Critically Analysing the Literature   69

7 Synthesising the Literature   90

8 Writing up Your Literature Review   111

9 Referencing and Plagiarism   119

10 What comes next?   129

Glossary   137

References   143

Index   151

Figures
and Tables

Figures

3.1	Example of Flowchart from Database Search	41
7.1	Example of a Forest Plot	102
7.2	Components of Meta-study	106

Tables

2.1	Two Approaches to Concept Analysis	24
4.1	Nursing, Health and Social Care Related Databases	54
4.2	Using Boolean Operators (CINAHL search undertaken 20 December 2011)	58
6.1	Credibility and Integrity Factors in a Quantitative Research Study	72
6.2	Credibility and Integrity Factors in a Qualitative Research Study	79
6.3	Integrity Factors in a Systematic Review	86
6.4	Analysing Non-research Literature	88
7.1	Example of Tabulation of Online Database Search	91
7.2	Summary Table – Example 1	92
7.3	Summary Table – Example 2	93
7.4	Example 1 of Summary Table for Systematic Reviews	94
7.5	Example 2 of Summary Table for Systematic Reviews	95
7.6	Example of Summary Table for Non-research literature	96
7.7	Example of Additional Information that May Be Presented	96
7.8	Methods for Synthesising Data	96
7.9	Example of Analysis in a Metasynthesis	97
7.10	Example of Synthesis: Identity and Coping Experiences in Chronic Fatigue Syndrome	105

About the Authors

Michael Coughlan is an Assistant Professor in the School of Nursing, Trinity College Dublin, where he has worked since 2002. He is a Registered Nurse Tutor and has been involved in nurse education for over 20 years. He has a wide experience in guiding and supervising students undertaking literature reviews and research studies at both an undergraduate and postgraduate level. His interests include research, and haematology and oncology nursing and he has a number of publications in these areas.
Qualifications: BNS, MEd., RPN, RGN, RNT.

Patricia Cronin is an Assistant Professor in the School of Nursing and Midwifery, Trinity College Dublin. She took up her post there in 2004 having worked at City University, London for the preceding 10 years. Her clinical background is in surgical and gastrointestinal nursing, which she teaches at undergraduate level. She has a special interest in enabling students to engage in research and theory and these areas from the focus of her postgraduate teaching. She has published widely, co-authoring two books and written book chapters and journal articles related to clinical skills, gastrointestinal nursing, research and theory.
Qualifications: PhD, MSc, BSc Nursing & Education, DipN (Lond), RN.

Frances Ryan is an Assistant Professor-Lecturer in General Nursing in the School of Nursing and Midwifery, Trinity College Dublin and has been there since 2002. She is a registered General and Children's Nurse and has worked extensively in the area of adult intensive care nursing. She is a Registered Nurse Tutor and has a Masters in Education. Her previous research has focused on empowerment in adult education. Her areas of teaching include interpersonal and communication skills, reflective practice in nurse education and research methodologies. She has published articles on research in the *British Journal of Nursing* and the *International Journal of Therapy and Rehabilitation* as well as co-authoring the chapter, 'Physical Health and Mental Health Nursing' (Morrissey et al., 2007, *Psychiatric/Mental Health Nursing – Concepts, Applications, Challenges*. Dublin: Gill and Macmillan). Her current area of research is concerned with palliative care and she has been awarded funding from the Irish Hospice Foundation to assist in the development of this project.

1

What is a Literature Review?

Introduction

The process of undertaking a literature review is an integral part of doing research. While this may be considered to be its primary function, the literature review is also an important tool that serves to inform and develop practice and invite discussion in academic work. Whatever its purpose, the task of doing a literature review is often viewed as an onerous and confusing one by students. The aim of this chapter is to provide you, the student, with a comprehensive understanding of what a literature review is and, equally, what it is not. It explores its purpose and relevance and the differences between the literature review and other forms of academic writing. The fundamental steps involved in undertaking a literature review will also be considered. Whether or not you have previously embarked on the literature review journey, this chapter is designed to help you understand the process and skills involved in navigating the literature and reaching your ultimate destination.

☑ Learning Outcomes ☑

By the end of this chapter you should be able to:

- explain what a literature review is.
- outline the differences between writing a literature review and writing an essay.
- describe the steps in undertaking a literature review.

What is a Literature Review? Beginning Your Journey

Whether it is for clinical or academic purposes (or your own innate curiosity!) it is important to understand what a literature review is before you start sourcing and immersing yourself in copious amounts of research and theoretical concepts. A literature review is a synopsis of other research. Moreover, it is a critical appraisal of other research on a given topic that helps to put that topic in context (Machi and McEvoy, 2009). A comprehensive review should provide the reader with a succinct, objective and logical summary of the current knowledge on a particular topic. Therefore, it is not an essay of one's own personal views and opinions. Similarly, it is not a series of quotes or lengthy descriptions of other people's work. Quite simply, the literature review provides a critical discussion on the topic of interest while pointing out similarities and inconsistencies in existing relevant literature. It is important to note that while a literature search is the means of helping you to unearth literature that is appropriate to your task in hand, a literature review is the process of critically evaluating and summarising that literature.

The Purpose of the Literature Review: The Question and Context

Conceptualising the Literature Review

Think of a topic that interests you in clinical practice. Imagine this as a wide-rimmed, intricate crystal vase that tapers to a very narrow stem. There are some imperfections in the crystal. The rim represents the body of knowledge surrounding your chosen topic, and the stem represents your ultimate research question. Imagine the vase as your literature review. What does it mean? What do you need to do?

In the above activity you have already embarked on the process of starting your literature review. By undertaking an initial, broad literature search and then review, you will eventually be at the stage of fine-tuning and narrowing down your research idea or question in the context of other literature. A thorough and critical review of the literature will enable you to do just that. It is important to mention here that some literature reviews are preceded by a pre-determined research question and, therefore, how and when they are conducted varies according to the type of approach used. For example, quantitative research studies are usually driven by the context of previous knowledge, with specific research questions in mind based on conducting an extensive literature review before data collection commences.

Qualitative studies typically adopt a less structured approach to doing a literature review at the outset. They may start with a broad research question or topic of interest that is refined and honed as data are collected. Therefore, while the literature may be consulted briefly at the outset, a more thorough and in-depth review is done based on emerging data rather than pre-existing knowledge. Whatever the approach, the purpose of the review is to provide an analysis and synthesis of all the available literature on a given subject in a critical fashion. This then allows for further understanding of the subject in the context of what is already known. Furthermore, it can lead to the development of new research questions. Using the analogy of the crystal vase, each individual piece of crystal (including the imperfections) fits with the others to make the vase whole and cannot be viewed in isolation. Similarly, for the literature review to be complete and comprehensive, it needs to be carried out and evaluated in light of all other relevant literature, in order to get the fullest picture possible.

The Importance of Reviewing the Literature

The importance of the literature review is directly related to its aims and purpose. Nursing and allied health disciplines contain a vast amount of ever increasing literature and research that is important to the ongoing development of practice. The literature review is an aid to gathering and synthesising that information. The purpose of the literature review is to draw on and critique previous studies in an orderly, precise and analytical manner. The fundamental aim of a literature review is to provide a comprehensive picture of the knowledge relating to a specific topic. For example, if one is proposing to undertake a research project, then the purpose of the literature review is to situate that project in its relevant context or background. It does this by drawing on previous work, ideas and information. In addition, a good review will extract and critically evaluate the pertinent findings and issues that have emerged from previous work (Hart, 2010). By doing so, it provides justification for the proposed research and demonstrates a thorough grasp of background knowledge. Going back to our analogy of the crystal vase, it is evident that some imperfections exist. These we can take to represent evidence that is not strong and cannot be viewed in isolation. To do so would give an incomplete picture. Therefore, the literature needs to be reviewed in the context of all other information relating to the topic. One single viewpoint or article will not give the full story and may serve to bias the review.

Box 1.1   Defining Your Research Question

In health and social sciences, research questions usually stem from practice and serve to inform and develop practice. Defining your question can be a difficult task. Think of a particular area of practice that interests you. Ask yourself what you know about it. Now think, what is it you want to find out? For example, you may have an interest in the impact of type II diabetes. Ask yourself, Why? What? Who? Where? How? Decide what your question is and keep close to it. Your literature review should proceed from the known to the unknown, guided by your research question.

The importance of the literature review cannot be overstated. It is the tool to advancing practice. Furthermore, it can help to inspire and generate new ideas by highlighting inconsistencies in current knowledge (Aveyard, 2010). Literature reviews are not undertaken solely for the purpose of doing research. They have an important function in evaluating current practice and making recommendations for policy development and change. They are also useful for exploring existing theoretical or conceptual frameworks concerning a given subject. Similarly, they facilitate the development of theoretical or conceptual frameworks through exploration and critical evaluation of existing knowledge. The manner in which the review is written is a crucial component of understanding what a literature review is and often poses the greatest challenge to students. Before we discuss the steps in undertaking a literature review we need to examine what differentiates it from other types of academic writing.

Essay Writing versus Writing a Literature Review

Essay writing is a process that communicates ideas to an intended reader, and is usually written according to pre-determined academic conventions. An essay may have many purposes but its basic format is structured as an introduction, main body and conclusion that convey information relating to the essay question. The question serves to focus and direct the student as to what is required in the essay. For example, the question may require the student to produce a general overview of a topic. On the other hand, the purpose of the essay may be to produce a specific analysis of a particular subject; therefore the question will be phrased differently. Words such as discuss, explain, describe, analyse and assess may be an integral part of the question and will determine what approach to writing should be adopted. In some instances, a particular topic may not have been assigned and, therefore, it is up to the student to decide the purpose of the essay and what they are trying to achieve – that is, is the purpose to inform or educate, or perhaps create a persuasive argument?

Common essay types include judgement essays, exploratory essays and reflective essays (Shields, 2010). Judgement essays typically defend a particular argument or viewpoint and attempt to persuade or convince the reader to adopt the writer's stance. Judgement essays are based on an evaluation of relevant evidence and theories surrounding a topic and are written with the intention of constructing a sound argument that defends the writer's viewpoint. The judgement essay requires the writer to produce a subjective account of an issue, based on a discussion and interpretation of existing evidence. In contrast, exploratory essays do not require the writer to adopt a particular stance. This type of essay is concerned with producing a reasoned explanation of a given subject or phenomenon. It explores an issue in a logical and thorough fashion and presents and explains factual information in a balanced manner, without defending a particular viewpoint. The exploratory essay is concerned with a review, comparison and discussion of theories relating to a specific subject area. Both judgement and exploratory essays require a level of critical analysis of the essay question (Shields, 2010). The reflective essay is based on the premise that learning occurs and is enhanced through reflection. While reflective essays require a format similar to other essays, this is typically less structured as reflection is personal to the writer and so the style and language used will differ from more formal essay writing. Reflective essays are not based on a question but tend to focus on description and analysis of a personal incident or experience with a view to learning from that event. While reflective essays are descriptive in nature, it is necessary to discuss relevant theories and concepts relating to the event in order to analyse it.

So what then of the literature review, and does it differ from other types of essay writing? There are some similarities. As when writing an essay, one needs to have a structure and focus when undertaking a literature review. There is a sequence of events that should be adhered to in order to create a comprehensive review. The style and language must adhere to academic convention. Sections need to be cohesive and flow logically. Concepts and theories should be compared and contrasted, grouped for similarities and inconsistencies. Evidence needs to be analysed and discussed in relation to its context and significance.

The difference between essay writing and writing a literature review is that while the purpose of essay writing is generally to discuss ideas with respect to the essay question, the aim of the literature review is to summarise and synthesise all that is published on a given topic. The literature review is undertaken to present results of research and key information in an objective and discursive manner. In contrast to the essay, the literature review should summarise the key concepts, theories and empirical studies while discussing their strengths and limitations. If this is done for the purposes of research, then it needs to be focused, in-depth and relevant to the research question. Critical discussion is a crucial component of writing a good review. A literature review is not a descriptive, exploratory essay. Similarly, unlike the judgement essay, it does not seek to defend a particular viewpoint, nor does it offer personal opinion or speculation, as does the reflective essay. It is not a criticism, but rather is a critical review that goes beyond description to the level of critique, analysis and synthesis. Writing a literature review can be considered difficult when one has been accustomed to essay-style writing. The basic structure of introduction, main body and conclusion still applies, with some specific additional steps that serve to further differentiate literature review writing versus essay writing.

Steps in Undertaking a Literature Review

A literature review is an essay of sorts; however, it tends to be more formulaic in nature. The key steps to undertaking any literature review firstly involve developing a structure for the review. This entails selecting the review topic, carrying out a literature search, reading, critiquing and analysing the literature, and finally writing the review. The approach to writing a literature review will vary slightly according to the type of review undertaken. For example, a systematic review will have a specific format that must be adhered to throughout (Cronin et al., 2008). The different types of literature review and their purpose will be discussed in detail in Chapters 2 and 3. Structuring the review so that it is presented in a clear, coherent and consistent manner is vital, and it is necessary to develop a framework for this before starting to write. A well-organised literature review will consist of an introduction, a main body that critiques the findings of previous work, addressing both theoretical and empirical literature, a discussion and a conclusion.

Selecting a topic to review is the first step in the process. Selecting a topic is guided by your overarching research objective or the problem you wish to explore. Carrying out a literature search involves using both primary and secondary sources, as well as theoretical or anecdotal papers relevant to the topic. The search strategy and terms used should be stated in order to provide evidence that the review was thorough and comprehensive. It is important to narrow down the review topic or research question to avoid generating overwhelming amounts of information. A general idea of the area of interest is a good starting point, but it is necessary thereafter to hone this to a specific aspect of interest in order to make the review manageable. Searching the literature effectively will enable you to do this. The importance of a thorough literature search cannot be overstated, as this will enable you to broaden your knowledge of your chosen topic. It also helps situate the research question in the context of existing knowledge. A comprehensive literature search facilitates better understanding and awareness of the appropriate approach for your own study (Ridley, 2008). Selecting a topic and the various approaches to literature searching are explored in depth in Chapter 4.

Searching and reading the literature is a continuous process in the early stages of doing a literature review. Reading will inform your searching and direct you to new areas to explore. Similarly, a thorough literature search will influence your research question and provide direction for your writing. At the preliminary reading stage, it is useful to summarise what you have read by note taking and keeping records of what sources of literature are pertinent for the review. This will help to focus the review, refine your own ideas and assist in the final write-up. Organising the literature for easy retrieval is an essential task that will also help in the writing-up stage. Chapter 5 examines strategies for reading and organising literature in more detail.

Analysis and synthesis are the next stages in the process of doing a literature review, and at this point all of the relevant information should have been gathered. Once an initial overview has been done, it is necessary to critique and critically analyse the literature in order to obtain a critical review of the content. When writing the final review it is important that key information is critically evaluated, rather than described. Evidence needs to be summarised and presented logically, comparing and contrasting findings, and offering new insights where possible. Chapters 6 to 8 discuss how to analyse, synthesise and write the review.

Box 1.2   Putting it Together

A checklist is useful to have when undertaking a literature review. In order to stay focused throughout the process, think about the following issues:

- Have you identified a specific research question?
- What type of literature review are you conducting?
- How will you conduct your literature search?
- What is the scope of your review? What type of publications will you use and from what discipline?
- Have you identified the type of literature that will help you address your research question?

- Has your literature search been extensive enough to include all relevant material? Has it appropriate breadth and depth?
- Have you critically analysed the literature and discussed its strengths and weaknesses?
- Have you identified conflicting findings and offered possible reasons?
- Is your literature review balanced and objective?
- Have you discussed the significance of the findings?
- Is your literature review written in a logical and succinct manner?
- Have you identified and discussed implications for practice and further research?

Summary

A literature review is a critical evaluation of extensive research and theory relating to a specific topic. It is the process of analysis and synthesis of previous work in order to produce a summary of the knowledge on that topic. It gives insights into the background and context of a proposed study and is a logical, coherent argument that arises from a critical analysis of the state of knowledge in a specific topic area. This chapter has addressed the concept of what the literature review is and its importance and relevance in practice and research. We have also explored how it differs from other forms of academic writing. The steps involved in undertaking a literature review have been outlined and discussed briefly.

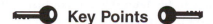 **Key Points**

- A literature review is a critical evaluation of knowledge of a topic.
- The literature review may be used as a basis for research, practice and policy development or academic purposes.
- The steps to undertaking a literature review involve selecting a topic and literature searching, reading and organising the literature, analysis and synthesis, and writing up the final review.

2

Types of Literature Review

Introduction

This chapter focuses on the various types of literature review that you may encounter when reading the literature, and it is important that you can distinguish between them for a number of reasons. First, in recent years there has been a noticeable increase in the terms that have been used to describe the 'literature review' and, to those of you who may be accessing academic literature for the first time, the discussion can be daunting and confusing in terms of differentiating between them. Second, throughout your undergraduate programme and beyond, being able to analyse and critique published literature is fundamental. Much has been written about how to do this in respect of research reports but there has been limited guidance on how to make a judgement about the quality of a literature review. However, with the advent and proliferation of what are termed systematic reviews, tools and guidance have been emerging, such as the Assessment of Multiple Systematic Reviews (AMSTAR) (Shea et al., 2007) and the Critical Appraisal Skills Programme (CASP) for Systematic Reviews (www. caspinternational.org). Nonetheless, it is suggested here that the ability to determine if a reviewer has conducted a 'good' review starts with determining if there is congruence between the type of review they said they were going to do and what they actually did. Third, in the event that you have to conduct a review, it is important that you have clear indicators of the requirements of your particular review.

This chapter begins with a brief outline of how the conceptualisation and categorisation of the literature review has developed. This is followed by an overview of the various types of literature review as well as offering some clarity around the use of terms. Examples are offered throughout to enhance understanding.

☑ **Learning Outcomes** ☑

By the end of this chapter you should be able to:

- explain the purpose of different types of literature review.
- describe the major differences between the various types of literature review.
- outline how the stated purpose of a literature review directs the type of review to be undertaken.

The Changing Literature Review

Traditionally, literature reviews have been seen as being embedded in the various stages of the development, conduct and reporting of a research study or as a vital part of an academic assignment. However, in recent decades several factors have combined to transform and expand their role and functions.

The Knowledge Explosion

The increasing sophistication of online technology and the advent of online databases have led to an explosion of available literature that is enormously beneficial when compared with the pre-electronic days that involved spending many hours in libraries searching catalogues, handsearching journals and photocopying material. However, for practitioners who are interested in a topic for whatever purpose, the sheer volume of available literature means that the business of discerning and subsequently assessing and judging it is complex. Moreover, busy practitioners may be time constrained or may not have the wherewithal to undertake the level of analysis required to determine the quality of a series of individual or discrete studies. Consider, for example, the individual skills you need just to be able to access material electronically. At the very least, you have to have some computer literacy and you have to be able to discern what are 'credible' sources of material. Despite the assumption that computer literacy is a universal skill, we have over our years in education met many students who are daunted by the prospect. We have also noted that many in the early stages of their education do not have the skills to discriminate between that which is considered an acceptable source of information or evidence and that which is not. If these issues are put in the context of limited time and resources, locating and retrieving the evidence can be an intimidating process, and that is before you even consider what you are going to do when you have collected the material.

ACTIVITY 2.1

Go to any well-known search engine and type in any of the following terms:

- postoperative pain.
- mobility assessment.
- assessment of swallowing.

Note how many 'hits' you get but also look at the sources of the material and see if you can judge whether or not they are 'credible'.

Evidence-based Practice

In the context of the information explosion and possible overload, Hamer and Collinson (2005) argue that it is almost impossible for healthcare practitioners to stay up to date. Yet we have a professional obligation to try to provide the best care possible based on the best available knowledge and evidence. The rise in the popularity of evidence-based healthcare (EBH) that corresponded with the ever-increasing availability of information is a reflection of this obligation. Early work in EBH was largely in the field of medicine and is important for this discussion in that the evidence-based medicine movement (EBM) promoted summarising the evidence from clinical research, thereby reducing the emphasis on 'unsystematic clinical experience and pathophysiological rationale' (Guyatt et al., 2004: 990). Evidence, in this sense, is seen to be external clinical evidence from systematic research. Because of this, a form of literature review known as the systematic review shot to prominence in the health sector.

It is important to note here that evidence-based medicine, or the more encompassing term of evidence-based practice (EBP) because the approach is not confined to medicine, incorporates more than identifying best evidence. It is about 'the conscientious, explicit, and judicious use of current best evidence in making decisions about the care of individual patients' (Sackett et al., 1996: 71). Muir Gray (2001) epitomises this as doing the right things for the right people at the right time where clinical expertise and consideration of the individual patient's needs, situation, rights and preferences are factors that influence whether the 'evidence' is applied. Therefore, good evidence is not the only determinant of the right thing to do, and issues such as patient empowerment, cost pressures, changing public expectations and political consensus complicate the translation of strong evidence into practice. Later in the chapter the significance of this will be demonstrated when considering various types of literature review.

Nonetheless, despite some detractors who claim EBM/EBP suppresses clinical freedom, there is now almost universal recognition from practitioners, managers and policy-makers that in order to deliver effective healthcare scientific evidence is an essential element. However, given the limitations identified above with the sheer volume of information and the skills and time needed to source and summarise the evidence the question is, how can practitioners determine what is best evidence?

In acknowledgment of this and in order to facilitate summarising evidence about the effectiveness of healthcare interventions, the Cochrane Centre in Oxford (now the UK Cochrane Centre (http://ukcc.cochrane.org/) was founded in 1992, and in the following year The Cochrane Collaboration (www.cochrane.org) was launched. Since then, it has become an internationally recognised organisation that has over 28,000 participants from more than 100 countries. See examples from their top 50 wide-ranging reviews in Box 2.1.

Box 2.1   Reviews from The Cochrane Collaboration

A critical assessment of any associations between green tea consumption and the risk of cancer incidence and mortality (Boehm et al., 2009).

[The choice of] first-line drugs for hypertension (Wright and Musini, 2009).

In recent years, the National Institute for Health Research (www.nihr.ac.uk) has funded the National Health Service (NHS) Centre for Reviews and Dissemination (CRD) (www.york.ac.uk/inst/crd/), which undertakes and disseminates the results of reviews that are of importance to the NHS. As with the Cochrane library, there are diverse examples in their databases (Box 2.2).

Box 2.2   Reviews from Centre for Reviews and Dissemination (CRD)

Music as a nursing intervention for postoperative pain: a systematic review (Engwall and Sorensen, 2009).

Artificial nutrition and hydration in the last week of life in cancer patients (Raijmakers et al., 2011).

Another organisation that has relevance for healthcare, but is not directly concerned with determining the effectiveness of clinical interventions, is the Evidence for Policy and Practice Information and Co-ordinating Centre (EPPI-Centre) (http://eppi.ioe.ac.uk/cms). The EPPI-Centre emerged from a project at the Social Science Research Institute in London that aimed to develop a database of evaluations of interventions in the fields of education and social welfare. Since its foundation, its work has expanded to include reviews in education and social policy, health promotion and public health, international development and participative research and policy. Some recent examples are cited in Box 2.3.

Box 2.3   Reviews from EPPI Centre

Children's views about obesity, body size, shape and weight (Rees et al., 2009).

The relationship between speech, language and communication difficulties (SLCD) and emotional and behavioural difficulties (EBD) in children of primary school age (5–12 years) (Law and Plunkett, 2009).

A further development was The Campbell Collaboration (www.campbellcollaboration.org), which followed the establishment of The Cochrane Collaboration and adopted its methodology to examine the effects of interventions in areas outside of health and incorporating broader public policy. Examples include a review of the research evidence on 'the effects of early family/parent training on child behaviour problems including anti-social behaviour and delinquency' (Piquero et al., 2008).

As can be seen from the brief overview of the organisations and centres that have emerged and developed in the last two decades, the concept of synthesised evidence has become a fundamental factor in clinical, healthcare, managerial, educational, social and public policy decision-making. As a result of these developments, conceptualisations of the literature review have expanded and changed irrevocably.

Primarily, this is because when these organisations set themselves the task of summarising the evidence from research they deemed it necessary to develop criteria for ensuring the quality, consistency and transparency of the review process. As a result, protocols were introduced into the world of literature reviewing and became the hallmark of the systematic review.

Hierarchies of Evidence

What is important in terms of literature reviewing is that these protocols not only determine how a review is to be conducted but dictate the type of primary study design that should be included. The belief is that some study designs produce more reliable results. Thus, there are hierarchies of evidence where some evidence is valued more highly, based primarily on the type of research used to generate it (Hamer and Collinson, 2005). For example, in healthcare research that examines the effectiveness of clinical interventions, the randomised controlled trial (RCT) is ranked as the 'gold standard' study design (see Box 2.4 for a definition). This is because the procedures adopted in undertaking RCTs attempt to minimise the effect of confounding factors with the result that the findings are more likely to represent the 'true effect' of the intervention (Evans, 2003). Although much has been written about the limitations of RCTs in evaluating healthcare interventions (see Parahoo, 2006: 450), they are still considered to be at the highest level of evidence.

Box 2.4   Definition of Randomised Controlled Trial

A simple definition of a randomised controlled trial is that it is an experiment for the purpose of testing the effectiveness of an intervention, for example a new medication. Those who are taking part are randomly assigned to either the intervention group (to receive the new medication) or the control group (not to receive the new medication). The results are compared between the two groups.

An outcome of these developments is that literature reviews themselves are now 'ranked', with systematic or protocol-driven reviews being most highly valued. It is argued that this is because the process of undertaking such a review is highly structured, logical and transparent, with all decisions being clearly explained throughout. Therefore, regardless of their underlying purpose, all literature reviews are now judged against the standard or benchmark of the systematic review. Even the literature review that you undertake on a topic for an assignment will likely incorporate elements of the systematic review process. To some extent, this has had implications for reviews that do not meet the criteria for a systematic review. For example, the 'traditional' (also variously described as 'narrative', 'descriptive', 'standard') review has seen its position eroded to a point where it is regarded by some as being the least structured and thereby the least significant. Moreover, the rapid rise of the systematic review has resulted in an associated growth of published literature reviews and with it a plethora of terms that are used to describe various 'types' of review (Box 2.5).

While this proliferation of all types of reviews has contributed to the development of more systematic and rigorous methods, Arksey and O'Malley (2005) argue that the labels appear to be applied loosely and there is a lack of consistency in terms of definition. In addition, there are a number of publications where the focus is on authors promoting the merits of their own approach. In some instances, rather than adding clarity, this merely serves to confuse the issue further. Therefore, when reading about each type of review presented in this chapter, you should consider the examples offered and reflect on whether the differences are apparent or whether you think the labels are merely a matter of semantics.

Box 2.5   Some Terms that Are Used to Describe Types of Literature Review*

- Narrative.
- Traditional.
- Descriptive.
- Standard.
- Integrative.

(Continued)

(Continued)

- Scoping.
- Qualitative.
- Concept analysis.
- Realist.
- Rapid evidence.
- Systematic.
- Meta-analysis.
- Meta-synthesis.
- Meta-summary.
- Meta-ethnography.

(*This list is not exhaustive or complete.)

Therefore, in this text we present the argument that all literature reviews share the fundamental characteristics of collecting, evaluating and presenting available evidence on a given topic. We also share Arksey and O'Malley's (2005) contention that there is no single type of 'ideal' literature review but a range of methods that need to be adopted appropriately depending on the focus of the review. Therefore, while some authors present reviews on a continuum from least to most systematic or structured in terms of their approach, we have chosen to present each as a discrete 'type'. Differences between each will be highlighted but comparisons in terms of their value are avoided.

Types of Literature Review

Traditional/Narrative Review

As indicated above, interchangeable terms that are used to describe this type of review include standard, traditional, narrative and descriptive. In this text, the term narrative is used for ease of description and because it is the term that appears most commonly in the literature.

Prior to the emergence of systematic reviews of interventions, the narrative review was the primary means by which literature on a given topic was presented. However, as outlined above, it is regarded by some as one that lacks any defined method for searching and retrieving the literature and is therefore described as being the least rigorous. While this may have been the case in the past, it is unlikely that you will see such reviews published as they will not meet the more systematic and rigorous methods that have evolved from the proliferation of all types of reviews (Whittemore and Knafl, 2005).

The increasing emphasis on reviews that are methodical means that the narrative review must, at least, meet the basic standard of having a clearly outlined method by which it was conducted. The result of these developments means that sometimes what are essentially narrative reviews are described in a publication title as 'systematic'.

This term may be used by the authors to indicate that the review was undertaken methodically rather than actually following a systematic review process.

Properly conducted narrative reviews remain a vital part of the science of any discipline. Overall, their aim is to identify, analyse, assess and interpret a body of knowledge on a topic. The particular focus and the breadth and depth of literature to be included in the review vary according to the context in which it is being conducted. For example, a literature review is a normal part of undertaking a research dissertation or thesis, and its function is to situate and justify the selection of the topic in the context of the existing literature. In funding proposals, reviews tend to present the current literature while also identifying gaps in existing knowledge. A narrative review may be presented also as a chapter in a book with the purpose of presenting the state of existing knowledge on a topic. It can be undertaken as a stand-alone, substantive review that is valuable in offering a connection between different aspects of a particular topic or even proposing a different or new interpretation of it. The narrative review is also the basis of many academic assignments and results in student learning through exploration of a specified topic.

Consequently, the topic areas for narrative reviews can vary from relatively broad to specific. In general, however, they are less precise than the type of question or problem that would be posed in any protocol-driven type of review. For example, Williams and Manias (2008) conducted a literature review on pain assessment and management in patients with chronic kidney disease. Although there was some specificity in respect of the focus on chronic kidney disease, pain assessment and management are very broad topics that resulted in literature being retrieved from a wide range of sources.

Because the focus is broader the type of literature sourced in a narrative review tends to be broad also. In Williams and Manias' review, the authors did not confine themselves to empirical research studies but included every type of publication that addressed pain and kidney disease or renal failure. These incorporated review and discussion papers as well as textbooks, and resulted in four renal textbooks and 93 articles being retrieved for full review. Of these, 12 were research papers using diverse methodologies and approaches relating to pain control in patients with chronic kidney disease. The key point here is that in a narrative literature review, you are not constrained by the type of literature you can use. However, it is fundamental that at the very least there is clarity about how you came to identify such literature and why you chose to include it.

For example, even when you are undertaking a literature review as part of an academic assignment you will be expected to outline the parameters you put in place when you searched the literature. These include delineating the databases you used, the key search terms you employed and how you combined them, the time limits you applied and any language restrictions you put in place. In addition, it is likely you will be expected to outline what you found, such as the volume and type of literature and how you undertook the subsequent analysis (e.g. thematic analysis – see Chapter 7) to arrive at the final selection. It is worth noting, however, that it is often the analysis and synthesis aspects of narrative reviews that are poorly developed. For those who wish to publish their reviews, it is unlikely that they will be accepted for publication unless they meet these parameters. Further details on these processes are addressed in Chapter 7.

Outlining the methods you adopted is also important because there is a risk of what is known as 'selection bias' where the reviewer only chooses literature that supports their standpoint. Nonetheless, the narrative review does not have to be a review of all the available literature and, in fact, it would be unrealistic to attempt to do so. What is fundamental is that the literature selected is relevant, that no key report is excluded and that the body of literature is adequately represented in the final review (Sandelowski, 2008). Therefore, many contemporary reviews tend to have a particular stance or focus that makes the review of the available literature more manageable (see Box 2.6).

Box 2.6   A Focused Narrative Review

Metastatic Breast Cancer Recurrence: A Literature Review of Themes and Issues Arising from Diagnosis (Warren, 2009)

As part of a larger study, Warren (2009) undertook a broad literature review with the purpose of identifying issues affecting women who had secondary breast cancer. As a result, she noted that while many studies examined quality of life in patients receiving a variety of treatments, little attention was given to the personal impact of recurrent disease. She conducted the review as follows:

Database Searches

- *Electronic databases*: CINAHL, Medline, AMED, British Nursing Index, PscyINFO, Cochrane Library from 1984 to January 2008.
- *Handsearches*: Journal contents pages/article reference lists.

Search Terms

Individually and in combination: 'recurrent', 'recurrence', 'cancer recurrence', 'metastatic breast cancer', 'advanced breast cancer', 'primary', 'initial', 'diagnosis'.

Findings

For this review, 23 articles were deemed relevant from the original 400 identified as part of the larger study. Using CASP as an analysis tool, the final selection consisted of 10 papers (three clinical reviews, and seven research studies – three qualitative, three quantitative and one mixed method).

Themes Identified

'Perceived difference in the impact of primary versus recurrent diagnosis', 'Previous experiences of cancer', 'Shock, surprise and the belief that risk of recurrence decreases over time', 'Loss of hope'.

Integrative Review

Another form of review that you may see in the literature is the integrative review. A brief overview is included here because it is likely you will encounter these in your reading and it is important to have some understanding in order that you can distinguish them from other types. Integrative reviews are, to some extent, a response to a perceived need for more systematic and rigorous approaches to reviewing the literature.

According to Broome (2000), an integrative review is one which summarises past research and draws conclusions on a given topic. In this definition the term research is interpreted in its broadest sense and literature that is sourced is not limited to empirical (primary) research studies. Theoretical or conceptual literature is also considered important (Whittemore and Knafl, 2005). Although proponents of the integrative review argue that there are some distinctions between it and a narrative review (Torraco, 2005), it can be difficult for the reader to distinguish between them, particularly where the latter has clearly stated and similar purposes. The purpose of an integrative review may be to provide a more comprehensive understanding of a concept or healthcare issue but it can also be used to create a new perspective or conceptualisation of a topic (Torraco, 2005). Thus, they have the potential to re-frame thinking or views of a phenomenon and contribute to the development of the knowledge base of a discipline by informing practice, policy and research (Whittemore and Knafl, 2005).

An example an integrative review is Whittemore's (2005) analysis of the concept of 'integration'. The purpose of this review was to update the definition and identify aspects of the experience of integration that are universal in relation to health, healing and nursing care. It is not essential at this time that you understand the concept of integration, but what is important is that Whittemore (2005) proposed that it is a significant aspect of healing and living with chronic illness. However, she recognised that there were inconsistencies in terms of how it was defined and how it was viewed theoretically. She proposed that through analysis of how integration is conceptualised in the theoretical literature and how it was explored in various research studies would add clarity to its meaning and advance understanding of how it contributes to healing, recovery and health. The conclusion of the review was presented diagrammatically as a model that depicted the process of integration.

The steps of an integrative review begin with the identification of a concept of interest. In Whittemore's case this was 'integration' but focused on how it related to health and illness. Clearly identifying the problem and purpose of the review is considered essential as it provides the focus and boundaries for all subsequent stages. As with any good review, the literature searching strategy should be rigorous as it helps prevent problems associated with incomplete searching and selection bias. Search strategies, inclusion and exclusion criteria, and results of searches must be clearly outlined.

Following extraction of the appropriate data (literature), decisions regarding evaluation of its quality are undertaken. This is particularly complex in any review, including an integrative review that draws on material from diverse sources such as empirical and theoretical literature. Moreover, it is likely that any integrative review will include research studies that are difficult to compare because they may have used a wide range of different methodologies or research designs. Both Broome (2000) and Whittemore and Knafl (2005) acknowledge this and recognise that this part of the process of undertaking an integrative review must be developed further. Nonetheless, some system for evaluating quality is essential for transparency regarding the outcomes of the review. Similarly, the process by which data analysis is undertaken can be complex and will depend on the type of literature that is being reviewed. Regardless, when reading the final report, you, as the reader, should be able to discern the approach taken. Read the précis of the integrative literature review in Box 2.7 and complete the associated activity.

Box 2.7   An Integrative Review

An Integrative Literature Review of Lifestyle Interventions for the Prevention of Type II Diabetes Mellitus (Madden et al., 2008)

Aim and Objectives

To critically appraise the literature on type II Diabetic Prevention Programmes (DPPs) to provide answers to the following questions:

1 What types of lifestyle interventions are used to prevent or delay the onset of type II diabetes?
2 Which types of lifestyle interventions produce the most effective results?
3 How likely are patients to persist in their adherence to lifestyle changes?

Inclusion/Exclusion Criteria

- Included primary research from peer-reviewed journals in English.
- Excluded studies where subjects had diabetes prior to intervention.
- Excluded studies that examined pharmacotherapy except the work of the Diabetes Prevention Program Research Group (DPPRG).

Search Strategy

- *Electronic databases:* Medline, CINAHL, Cochrane Databases of Systematic Reviews from 1996–2007.
- *Reference lists:* from retrieved articles.

Search Terms

'diabetes prevention programme', 'type II diabetes', 'prevention', 'prevention programmes'.

Findings

- Electronic database search found 85 scholarly articles.
- Handsearch of reference lists identified 30 articles.

Analysis

- Application of inclusion and exclusion criteria eliminated 94 articles.
- Assessment of abstracts left 12 studies from 8 journals.

Themes Identified

'types of interventions', 'most effective interventions', 'adherence'.

Examine the information provided in each aspect of Madden et al.'s (2008) integrative review and answer the following questions:

- Are the aims and objectives of the review clear?
- Are the inclusion and exclusion criteria appropriate?
- Is the search strategy clearly outlined?
- Do the search terms used help achieve the aims and objectives of the review?
- Have the authors outlined how they evaluated the literature?
- Do the authors outline how they arrived at the themes for the subsequent presentation of findings?

How do you think this example differs from the one by Warren (2009) cited in Box 2.6?

Scoping Review

Although they have been used for a number of years across a range of academic disciplines, the scoping review is a relatively new phenomenon in healthcare. In the literature you will also find them described variously as 'scoping studies', 'rapid scoping reviews' and/or 'scoping projects' (Davis et al., 2009). Davis et al. (2009) suggest also that scoping reviews/studies are poorly defined and they vary considerably in terms of their aims, the process by which the review is conducted and their methodological rigour. Usually, however, they consist of one or more discrete components, the most common of which is that they are non-systematic reviews, that is, they are not driven by a pre-determined protocol. Other noteworthy elements are that they may include consultations with stakeholders and literature mapping, conceptual mapping and/or policy mapping (Anderson et al., 2008). Again, it is a good idea to have some idea of what these reviews entail as it is likely you will come across them in your reading.

According to Arksey and O'Malley (2005: 21), there are four common reasons why a scoping study might be undertaken and these have been incorporated into key criteria for the commissioning of a scoping study by the NIHR Service Delivery and Organisation Research and Development programme (SDO Programme) (see Box 2.8).

Box 2.8   Reasons for Undertaking a Scoping Review/Study

- To 'map' the extent, range and nature of research activity in an area of study. In this type of scoping, the research may not be described in detail but might include mapping of concepts, policies, evidence and/or user views (separately or in combination).
- To determine the feasibility of undertaking a full systematic review or further empirical research. Feasibility is about determining if there is sufficient literature to undertake a systematic review or even if they have already been conducted.

(Continued)

(Continued)

- To summarise and disseminate research findings to policy-makers, practitioners and consumers.
- To identify gaps in the current research literature. In this type of scoping study, conclusions are drawn regarding the overall state of research activity in a particular area of study.
- To develop methodological ideas and/or theoretical approaches best suited to future research studies of a particular topic.
- To clarify conceptual understanding of a topic where definitions are unclear or where there is lack of agreement.
- To advise on and justify further research studies.
(Arksey and O'Malley, 2005; Anderson et al., 2008)

As is evident from Box 2.8, the reasons for undertaking a scoping review are diverse and there is considerable variety in terms of both the breadth and depth of literature extracted. It is also worth noting that scoping can be part of a preliminary investigation into an area or may be a stand-alone project. In healthcare, their ultimate aim is to facilitate asking the right questions in the context of health service organisation and management, healthcare practice and policy, and determining the research agenda in particular areas. They have been found to be particularly useful in identifying services that are available for discrete groups in the population (Anderson et al., 2008). However, it is important to emphasise that scoping reviews are not appropriate for answering clinical questions (CRD, 2009).

Given the wide range of functions that come under the umbrella term of scoping review/study it is difficult to outline in any definitive way the steps that should be followed. However, Arksey and O'Malley (2005) proposed a methodological framework (see Box 2.9) for conducting a scoping study with the intention of assuring a rigorous and transparent process.

Box 2.9   Methodological Framework for Conducting a Scoping Review

1 Identify the research question.
2 Identify the relevant studies.
3 Select the studies.
4 Chart the data.
5 Collate, summarise and report the results.
6 Optional stage: Consultation exercise.
(Arksey and O'Malley, 2005: 22)

Identifying the research question or focus of the review is the first step that enables the reviewers to define which aspects of the research are deemed most important. These subsequently guide the choice of search strategies. The CRD (2009) assert that the search strategy in a scoping review should be as extensive as possible with the purpose of identifying all relevant literature. Because of the complexity of the processes, it is recommended that a scoping review is undertaken by a multidisciplinary team rather than an individual. Searches should include a range of relevant databases, handsearching and efforts to seek unpublished literature by, for example, contacting established organisations, and via networks and conference materials. Initial search terms and strategies may be revisited as the reviewers become familiar with the literature.

As with all types of review, parameters for searching are decided at the outset, particularly in terms of time limits and language. Other aspects, such as budget and time constraints, may also limit the comprehensiveness of the review. In selecting studies, inclusion and exclusion criteria are developed but this may be after the initial search of the literature has taken place.

Data are usually charted according to an analytical framework that facilitates sorting the material into relevant themes. Collecting standard information such as authors, year of publication, aim, methods, study populations, intervention type, outcome measures and results is an example of one such framework. Following charting of the data, collating, summarising and reporting of the results are undertaken. These are often configured around the themes that have emerged from the review. This stage of the process is complex, time consuming and laborious given the breadth of literature sourced and the likelihood that the reviewer will still have a large amount of material to present.

An important factor is that scoping studies provide a descriptive account of the available research. They do not attempt to formally appraise the quality of the evidence in primary research reports. Neither do they make recommendations from the evidence about what is the most effective type of intervention. However, Arksey and O'Malley (2005) caution against assuming a scoping study is an easy alternative. There is the potential to generate a large number of studies that include a disparate number of designs and methodologies, and reviewers have to have the ability to analyse and present them in a coherent way.

A final optional step in a scoping review is consultation. Many contemporary scoping studies that are concerned with the identification of research priorities include consultation with stakeholders. Stakeholder consultation is an important element in contributing to service development and promoting user involvement in research (Anderson et al., 2008). See Box 2.10 for an example of a scoping review.

Box 2.10   A Scoping Review

Housing and dementia care – a scoping review of the literature (O'Malley and Croucher, 2005).

Research Question

What is known about housing and care provision for older people with dementia? (O'Malley and Croucher, 2005).

(Continued)

(Continued)

Aim

To describe the evidence base with regard to housing provision for elderly people with dementia with the aim of identifying gaps in existing knowledge.

Inclusion/Exclusion Criteria

- Included studies of housing and accommodation in relation to dementia in the UK since the early 1980s.
- Included overseas research that illuminates issues missing from the UK research agenda.
- Excluded non-empirical studies, theses, book reviews, commentaries, policy analyses.

Search Strategy

- *Electronic databases*: The Cochrane Library, MEDLINE, Social Science Citation Index, DH Data, HELMIS, The King's Fund, Sociological Abstracts, SIGLE (for grey literature), PsycINFO.
- *Websites*: of key mental health organisations.
- *Handsearches*: of main journals.
- *Bibliographies*: of located studies.

Search Terms

All main terms associated with the medical definition of 'dementia' with a combination of 'housing', 'long-term care', 'accommodation', 'residential', 'home care', 'continuing care', 'adult placement', 'group homes'.

Literature Located

- Identified 1675 references.
- Read 265 reports in detail.

Included 175 studies and reports in the final review.

Analysis

- Narrative synthesis included a description of the study and the findings. Gaps in the evidence were also noted.
- Thematic analysis according to type of accommodation or setting (own home/other family home, sheltered housing, very sheltered housing, long-stay residential care, end-of-life care).
- Accommodation subsequently classified as 'ordinary/domestic', 'special/collective' settings.

Findings

- Exposition of the 'ordinary/domestic' and 'special/collective' themes and sub-themes.
- Research gaps and methodological issues identified.

Concept Analysis

There has been a considerable amount of concept analysis work undertaken in healthcare in the last decade, particularly in the disciplines of nursing and midwifery. Concepts are mental images of phenomena, and it is through language that we give labels to these mental images in order that we can communicate with each other. For example, when we say the word 'horse', each of us has an image of what a horse looks like. It is through our experiences, perceptions and learning that we come to equate the mental image with the label 'horse'. However, language is complex and contextual and the meaning of a word can change over time, from one group to another or from one geographic area to another. Whilst the image of a horse may be reasonably universal there are many other concepts that are not as concrete, and meaning is only understood by the context in which the word is used. Many of the concepts in use in healthcare are what are known as behavioural concepts that are concerned with understanding health and illness experiences (Cronin et al., 2010). Examples include phenomena such as coping, self-care, suffering, hope, reassurance, anxiety, adherence, compliance and concordance. Imagine that a patient is about to have surgery and you determine from their behaviour and responses that they are anxious. As a result, you perceive that they need reassurance. Your mental image of both anxiety and reassurance will ultimately determine how you respond to the patient in question. It may well be an appropriate response on your part, but difficulties may arise when another person responds in another way because their understanding of the meaning of anxiety and reassurance is different, which can result in a lack of consistency in the standard and quality of care being delivered.

Make a list of concepts that are used in practice where you think there may be a lack of clarity.

Outline your reasons why you think such a lack of clarity may pose problems.

ACTIVITY 2.3

This lack of consistent understanding of a concept and its use in practice or research are the main reasons for undertaking a concept analysis. Simply stated, concept analysis is a method by which concepts that are of interest to any discipline are examined in order to clarify their characteristics, thereby achieving a better understanding of the meaning of that concept (Cronin et al., 2010).

Clear methodologies for undertaking concept analysis have evolved, and the most popular and most cited methods are outlined in Box 2.11. Although there are additional methods that include a 'fieldwork' stage, the focus here is on stand-alone concept analysis methods that are literature review based. Although a detailed discussion of the methods outlined in Table 2.1 is outside the scope of this book, some points regarding concept analysis are worth noting.

The concept selected for analysis should be relevant for practice and/or the research of the discipline. There should also be some ambiguity or lack of consensus as to its meaning or use within the context in which it is to be used. For example, in general usage most people will have an understanding of the concept of 'fatigue'. However,

Table 2.1   Two Approaches to Concept Analysis

Walker and Avant's method (2011)	Rodgers' Evolutionary method (2000)
1 Select a **concept**.	1 Identify the concept of interest and associated expressions (including surrogate terms).
2 Determine the aims or purpose of analysis.	
3 Identify **all uses** of the concept that you can discover.	2 Identify and select an **appropriate realm** for data collection.
4 Determine the **defining attributes**.	3 **Collect** relevant data.
5 Identify a **model** case.	4 **Analyse** the data.
6 Identify **borderline, related, contrary, invented and illegitimate** cases.	5 Identify an **exemplar** of the concept.
7 Identify **antecedents and consequences**.	6 Identify **implications,** for further development of the concept.
8 Define **empirical referents**.	

it has emerged in recent years that 'fatigue in chronic illness' is ill defined and has different characteristics from those which occur as a normal aspect of living. See Box 2.11 for McCabe's (2009) example of a concept analysis of fatigue in children with long-term conditions.

As with other types of literature review, a clear search strategy must be devised and explained, and all uses of the concept (physical, psychological, social) identified. This is important as the literature in a concept analysis will include sources such as dictionaries, thesauruses, the media, history and popular literature as well as discipline and non-discipline specific publications. This stage is likely to produce large amounts of data, particularly if the concept is in use in a variety of settings or disciplines. For example, the use of fatigue is not confined to healthcare and is also a key concept in areas such as sport and engineering.

Regardless of the method being used, the next stages involve review, analysis and synthesis of the literature to identify characteristics of the concept that appear repeatedly. This is a difficult and time-consuming process that generally follows a thematic analysis approach (see Chapter 7) where recurring themes are identified. At the same time, analysts are expected to derive antecedents and consequences of the concept. Antecedents are those things that cause the concept to happen, and consequences are what occur as a result of the concept (see Box 2.11).

Where concept analysis differs notably from other types of review is that, following analysis and synthesis of the literature, a model case or exemplar is presented to illustrate a pure example of the concept. It can be drawn from real life, found in the literature or in some instances constructed by the analyst.

Subsequent steps vary according to the method being used. For example, Walker and Avant (2011) argue that identifying 'other' cases that are not pure examples of the concept help to illustrate the differences between it and other concepts that may be related or similar, whereas Rodgers (2000) does not advocate this. Walker and Avant (2011) also promote identifying empirical referents, which are explicit criteria that show the concept exists. This can be in the form of an instrument that measures the concept. For example, in McCabe's (2009) concept analysis this would be an instrument to quantify the existence of fatigue in children with long-term conditions. Empirical referents are used as a basis for undertaking research.

Concept analysis is not for the faint-hearted as it is a lengthy process and can be frustrating due to the task of dealing with potentially vast amounts of literature. More recent analyses have tended to be more context specific, such as in McCabe's analysis, not only because it is recognised that the appearance of a concept may differ depending on the situation in which it is being considered but also because it reduces the amount of literature that has to be sourced. Nonetheless, another analyst might arrive at different outcomes because of the potential variation in the literature sourced and the level of critical thinking and analytical skills of the reviewer (Cronin and Rawlings-Anderson, 2004). Outcomes of concept analysis are always tentative as concepts change and develop with use or as practice situations change. A good example of this is Bissonette's (2008) analysis of the concept of 'adherence', in which she attempted to identify how and if the concept differed from the previously used concept of 'compliance'.

Box 2.11   A Concept Analysis

Fatigue in children with long-term conditions: an evolutionary concept analysis (McCabe, 2009).

Concept of interest

Fatigue in children with long-term conditions.

Aims

- To identify gaps in knowledge.
- To provide a clear definition of the concept.
- To clarify the current status of the concept and its use.

Surrogate terms

- Energy/Vitality.
- Tiredness.

Data sources

1 *Electronic databases*: CINAHL, Medline, PsychINFO.
2 Confined to English language from 1985 to 2007.
3 Five additional sources identified during review.
4 *Key words*: 'fatigue', 'child', 'childhood', 'adolescent', 'tiredness', 'fatigue syndrome'.

Literature retrieved

- CINAHL and Medline references (346).
- PsychINFO references(145).

(Continued)

(Continued)

Final sample

Sixty-two papers and two book chapters:

- Nursing references (34).
- Medical references (11).
- Psychology references (19).
- Research reports (43).
- Review papers (18).
- Expert opinions (3).

Data analysis

Thematic analysis with coding for attributes, antecedents, consequences, definitions, related concepts and surrogate terms.

Antecedents

- Imbalance in 'healthy routine' (nutrition, sleep, physical activity).
- Physiological disequilibrium.
- Stress, worry and fear.

Attributes

- Feeling of physical and emotional exhaustion.
- Decreased energy.
- Co-morbid pain or painful syndromes.
- Persists over time.
- Impacted by developmental stage.

Consequences

- Inability to engage in usual activities.
- Necessary to devise strategies to replenish or restore energy.
- Altered mood.
- Sleep disturbances.
- Social relationships impacted.
- School attendance/academic achievement.
- Negative quality of life.

Exemplar

No exemplar identified in this analysis.

Definition

A subjective experience of tiredness or exhaustion that is multidimensional and includes physical, mental and emotional aspects (McCabe, 2009).

Recommendations

- Ongoing international study to explore the experience of fatigue in children and advance understanding of the concept.
- Further exploration of the mechanism of fatigue in children so that appropriate interventions can be devised.
- Accurate measures of fatigue (behavioural and physiological).

Realist Review

Realist reviews (sometimes referred to as realist synthesis) have emerged in recognition of the complexity of healthcare interventions and the realisation that what is deemed to be the most effective intervention might work differently or not at all depending on the situation or circumstance in which it is being implemented. Social, environmental, economic and individual factors can all influence the effectiveness of an intervention and the focus of realist review is to examine these factors.

Realist review was developed originally for complex social interventions to examine how context influences the relationship between an intervention and its outcome. This is represented sometimes as context–mechanism–outcome (C–M–O) and asks how given contexts (C) have influenced or interfered with mechanisms (M) to generate the observed outcome(s) (O) (Greenhalgh et al., 2011). It focuses essentially on discovering what works, how it works, for whom it works, to what extent it works and under what conditions (Pawson et al., 2005). To date, much of the focus of realist reviews is in the areas of health policy and practice.

A realist review to understand the efficacy of school feeding programmes (Greenhalgh et al., 2007) is presented in Box 2.12 to provide an illustration of how such a review may be undertaken. As with all types of literature review, the realist review should begin with a clear question. However, this is not necessarily fixed and can be amended or additional questions can emerge as the data (literature) is retrieved and analysed. Sometimes, it may be appropriate to undertake a preliminary search of the literature to identify its nature and scope before finally deciding on the review questions (Mays et al., 2005).

Greenhalgh et al.'s (2007) realist review evolved from a Cochrane review of school feeding programmes for disadvantaged children, which included trials that spanned five continents and eight decades. Given that the Cochrane review identified that there was considerable variation in the designs of the trials, the educational settings in which the programmes were implemented as well as notable differences in the prevailing social, economic and political contexts, it was determined that knowing that the programmes worked was not sufficient. In order for policy-makers to decide which type of intervention should be implemented, it was deemed important to examine the trials in further detail to identify the factors that determined success or failure.

An important difference between realist and other types of review is the role of theory or mechanisms that underpin the types of interventions. The realist reviewer approaches the literature with the intention of searching for theories of why an intervention may work and why things went wrong (Pawson et al., 2005). Simply stated, this is about identifying the basis for believing a particular intervention will be successful. At this stage of the process the review team undertakes a comprehensive examination of theories underpinning the intervention being studied following which a list or subset of theories to be tested should be drawn up. Once this process is complete, the search for empirical evidence commences.

In the cited example, the literature for the review had already been determined by that which had been retrieved for the Cochrane review (Kristjansson et al., 2007). However, realist reviews will normally draw from a wide variety of research designs about the process of implementing the intervention. As with all reviews, the search strategies and retrieval mechanisms, including inclusion and exclusion criteria, must be rigorous and transparent. Mays et al. (2005) suggest that reviewers need to be fully conversant with the subject matter to ensure all pertinent search terms are included.

The synthesis stage is highly complex because of the variety of literature that is generally included and the need to evaluate the evidence with the purpose of judging the integrity with which each theory was tested. The reviewers should consider that the focus is not on the topic *per se* but on whether or not the study addressed the theory being tested (Pawson et al., 2005). Thus, the relative contribution of each source is assessed, explained and a judgement is made.

In Greenhalgh et al.'s (2007) study, for example, nine of the trials reviewed were based on the theory that school feeding corrects overt nutritional deficiencies, which then improves brain growth and performance. When identifying why a school programme did not work, the team concluded that the commonest reason for failure was a misguided theory, such as correcting a nutritional deficiency that did not exist.

The outcome of a realist review is not a final judgement on what works but is a revision about how it was thought the intervention would work (Pawson et al., 2005). This may result ultimately in changes to programmes in given settings. For example, one recommendation from Greenhalgh et al.'s (2007) review was that school feeding programmes should concentrate on children with documented nutritional deficiencies (see Box 2.12).

In keeping with many of the types of review outlined in this chapter, a realist review is a difficult undertaking. The reviewers must have a sound knowledge of the subject matter as well as an understanding of the issues that are of concern to policy-makers. In addition, reviewers need to have a deep-seated knowledge of research appraisal and skills of synthesis to ensure the rigour of the process. Given these factors and the possibility that review will involve a vast array of literature, it is unlikely that it would be attempted by an individual.

Box 2.12   A Realist Review

Realist Review to Understand the Efficacy of School Feeding Programmes (Greenhalgh et al., 2007)

Aim

To examine trials identified in a Cochrane review to establish aspects of school feeding programmes that determine success or failure.

Cochrane Review Search Strategy

- *Electronic databases*: CENTRAL (2006 Issue 2), MEDLINE (1966–May 2006), EMBASE (1980–May 2006), PsycINFO (1980–May 2006), CINAHL (1982–May 2006).
- *Handsearches*: of reference lists and key journals.
- Grey literature (Greylit network).
- Experts in the field, e.g. UNICEF.

Inclusion/Exclusion Criteria

- Included randomised controlled trials (RCTs), non-randomised controlled clinical trials (CCTs), controlled before and after studies (CBTs), interrupted time series studies (ITSs).
- Included children and adolescents in any country, aged 5–19 who attended primary or high school.
- Included children classified as being disadvantaged by defined criteria – for example children from economically marginalised or disadvantaged areas.
- Excluded children from urban areas with a large proportion of high socio-economic status (SES).
- Included interventions that were meals or snacks administered in a school setting.

Literature Retrieved

- Eighteen studies – seven RCTs, nine CBAs, two ITSs.

Realist Review Process

- Each trial reviewed individually for interaction between C–M–O.
- Reviewed across trials for patterns and idiosyncrasies.
- Synthesised key findings using a narrative and interpretive approach.

Results of Synthesis

Four broad areas relevant to the analysis were identified:

- historical context of school feeding programmes.
- theories to explain the success of particular programmes.
- theories to explain the failure or qualified success of particular programmes.
- measurement issues.

Outcomes

- Concentrate school feeding on pupils with documented nutritional deficiencies.
- A development phase (working with the local community to optimise and pilot the intervention) should be in place before the programme is tested in an experimental trial.
- In situations of absolute poverty, severely malnourished children may not benefit from school feeding programmes.

Systematic Review

Discussion of the systematic review in this chapter is limited to an outline of its tenets as further detail on the process of undertaking such a review is presented in Chapter 3. Summarised evidence about a particular intervention and its effectiveness has become an invaluable source of information for practitioners and decision-makers. Traditionally, as stated earlier in the chapter, systematic reviews have been concerned with reviews of effectiveness of interventions – that is, answering questions about 'what works' (CRD, 2009). They are generally classed as 'research on research' or secondary research because they do not collect new data but use the findings from previous research (Maxwell, 2006; Parahoo, 2006). Thus, most systematic reviews have the prefix 'meta', meaning 'after' or 'beyond', to indicate that they are second-order – that is, they come after and are based on previous or first-order studies (Zhao, 1991; 378). Systematic reviews are most likely to be undertaken when uncertainty exists regarding an intervention and the primary studies on the topic may have conflicting or disparate findings. The findings from the studies are pooled and analysed, and conclusions are drawn about the overall strength of the evidence.

The systematic review differs essentially from other types of literature review in that its methodology is explicit and precise. It follows a clearly outlined protocol that is standardised and replicable, thereby ensuring the quality, consistency and transparency of the review process. A further important feature is that the protocol, including decision-making in terms of what studies are eligible for inclusion, is normally constructed before the review is begun. Recently, however, it has been acknowledged that in some instances a more emergent or iterative process may be appropriate in some situations, but which is still clear and rigorous. Explicit criteria are used to judge the quality of the studies being reviewed and only those that are deemed to be of high quality are included. This process assists with reducing bias, thereby enhancing the reliability of the conclusions drawn.

Originally, the systematic review in healthcare was limited to undertaking a review of the findings of research from RCTs as they are considered to be at the highest level of evidence. However, within the systematic review community, there has been a notable shift and the boundaries of what is accepted as meeting the criteria for a systematic review have changed. This is because there is increased recognition that not all healthcare questions can be addressed by RCTs. In many instances, either RCTs do not exist or they would be an inappropriate approach to address the review question.

The outcome of this increased recognition is that the logic of the systematic review process has been extended to include a greater variety of research questions, types of evidence, range of research designs and methods for synthesising the evidence (EPPI, 2010). For example, recent developments have examined the impact of data from qualitative research and the expansion of the systematic review to include such data.

A further development has been the emergence of the systematic review of reviews. With the rapidly expanding number of systematic reviews, there may be situations where decision-makers are faced with more than one review on a topic or where there are questions regarding the quality and scope of the original review. As a result, systematic reviews of systematic reviews are now being conducted. Whilst the protocol and process are similar to that of an original systematic review, the literature sourced is confined to systematic reviews.

Summary

This chapter has outlined the various types of literature review you may encounter when examining published literature as part of your academic work, when exploring an issue related to your clinical practice or as part of the process of preparing a research proposal of your own. The types of review presented in this chapter are commonly published in academic journals but, as indicated earlier, this is not an exhaustive list as the range is ever expanding. The world of literature reviewing has become far more complex because of the recognised need to synthesise the increasingly vast amounts of available information and knowledge on a wide variety of topics. The advent of protocol-driven reviews as a means to manage this has resulted in a drive for more rigorous and systematic approaches to undertaking literature reviews. However, this has resulted in much debate and discussion about the merits or otherwise of these and non-protocol driven reviews such as the traditional, narrative review. It has been demonstrated also that undertaking a 'good' review is a difficult and time-consuming endeavour and many of the types presented here are likely to be beyond the scope of individual students and practitioners. Nonetheless, as a result of reading this chapter you should have a better understanding of the key, distinguishing features of the various types of literature review.

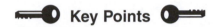

Key Points

- There is no single type of 'ideal' literature review but a range of methods that need to be adopted appropriately depending on the focus of the review.
- All literature reviews share the fundamental characteristics of collecting, evaluating and presenting available evidence on a given topic.
- In recent decades, factors such as the knowledge explosion, evidence-based practice and hierarchies of evidence have combined to transform and expand the role and function of the literature review.
- Systematic or protocol-driven reviews are valued most because the process of undertaking such a review is highly structured, logical and transparent.
- The advent of systematic or protocol-driven reviews has seen the position of the traditional or narrative review eroded, which is regarded by some as being the least structured and thereby the least significant.
- All literature reviews are now judged against the standard or benchmark of the systematic review with the result that all are likely to incorporate elements of the systematic review process.
- The rapid rise of the systematic review has resulted in an associated growth of published literature reviews and a plethora of terms that are used to describe various 'types' of review.
- The range of types of literature review is ever expanding in keeping with the various purposes for which they are being developed.
- Undertaking a 'good' literature review can be a difficult and time-consuming process and is one that requires the reviewer to develop skills in selecting, retrieving, organising and analysing a body of literature.

3

Systematic Review

Introduction

In the previous chapter an outline of the tenets of systematic review was presented in order to enable you to begin to discern how it differs from other types of literature review. This chapter develops these principles further and presents the process of conducting such a review. It is worth mentioning, however, that it is unlikely that you will be undertaking a systematic review as part of your undergraduate study as the process is complex and demanding. For the most part they are conducted in teams and can take a year or more to complete. Nonetheless, when you are searching the literature you will almost certainly source articles or publications that are entitled systematic review. It is important, therefore, that you have an understanding of what they are in order to be able to appraise them and determine if they meet the explicit criteria to be termed as such.

The focus of this chapter is an exploration of the systematic review methodology. As discussed in the previous chapter, a systematic review is a process whereby evidence from previously conducted, primary studies related to a particular topic is re-analysed and synthesised (Parahoo, 2006: 134). An important point is that systematic reviews are research studies and like all research enquiries they require an explicit and transparent methodology, which in turn facilitates the aim of reaching an unbiased conclusion (Engberg, 2008).

It is important to reiterate the point made in Chapter 2 that the systematic review is evolving and the types of questions being addressed and the methods for synthesising the evidence from a wide range of study designs have expanded (EPPI, 2010). This has generated some debate about whether a synthesis can be described as a systematic review if it is not a traditional review of effectiveness of interventions. What has emerged from these discussions is a sort of consensus that what makes a systematic review systematic is the use of a protocol that uses an explicit and transparent method. This means that not all reviews that are classed as systematic review follow the same synthesis method. For example, those that are undertaking systematic reviews of effectiveness of interventions will generally progress in a linear way through the recognised stages of study identification, quality assessment and synthesis. Others, such as those that use mixed or qualitative data, may adopt a more emergent approach that does not follow these stages exactly. Importantly, qualitative research is not a single method but a catch-all for a variety of study designs and data collection methods that are framed by diverse philosophical and theoretical perspectives. The result is that a number of methods for synthesis have been developed and are still evolving. Nevertheless, what is fundamental to all systematic reviews is that the authors explicate the process in order that readers can determine if the review has been undertaken rigorously in accordance with their declared approach. It is important when reading this chapter to keep these points and variations in mind.

☑ **Learning Outcomes** ☑

By the end of this chapter you should be able to:

- describe what is meant by a systematic review.
- outline the steps involved in conducting a systematic review.
- explain variations in the steps of the systematic-review process.

The Review Protocol

Preparing the review protocol is perhaps the most important part of conducting a systematic review because the thoroughness of the planning and preparation will ensure the process remains rigorous. The review protocol is similar to a research proposal produced prior to commencing a primary study in that it details the purpose of the review, presents the formulated question and objectives, outlines the processes for searching the literature, assessing and interpreting the data and presenting and disseminating the results. Although a protocol is developed in detail in advance of conducting the review, modifications are possible and may even be essential to ensure the findings are of value. Should changes be deemed necessary, these must be detailed in the final report.

Background

Prior to developing the protocol, it is important to address some background considerations. The primary consideration is to determine if the review is necessary. This includes situating the review and offering justification for why it needs to be undertaken. This will often be in relation to the potential significance and implications for clinical practice. Determining if the review is necessary also involves undertaking a search of the literature to see if the same or a very similar review has been completed already. This is referred to sometimes as a scoping review or scoping search (see Chapter 2). Reviews may exist on the topic but may not be of good quality or may require updating if they were conducted some time ago. If a good-quality review was conducted recently then there is little merit in doing another. In this instance, the reviewer could change the focus of the review question to include a different population, intervention or outcome. It is also worth noting that a scoping search may identify that there is no research available on the topic and therefore a systematic review will not be feasible.

A further background consideration is deciding about the team or panel to be involved in the review. As indicated in the introduction, systematic reviews are often undertaken in teams. These teams can comprise an expert panel or critical colleagues and/or service-users, depending on the research question (Bettany-Saltikov, 2012). Prior to commencing the review decisions regarding the composition of the team should be made. It is possible however, to undertake a systematic review individually, say as part of a dissertation, but the role of your supervisor is crucial in terms of providing advice and guidance to ensure the process is as valid and unbiased as possible.

Review Question, Aim, Objective

The first step in undertaking a systematic review is to identify a researchable question on a selected topic. As with any research study, the topic or research question can be generated from a number of sources. It may arise from a problem identified in clinical practice; it may be generated from an identified knowledge gap or may emerge from the existence of inconsistent or contradictory findings from individual studies. Systematic reviews are also commissioned by funding bodies where there are defined research priorities.

Review questions can be broad or narrow. Questions that focus on general management of a disease may be broad, whilst those that focus on the effectiveness of a particular intervention on a particular population or subset thereof may be narrow. However, if a question is very broad, it is often necessary to break it down further into more specific questions. For example, in the review presented in Box 3.1, the objective would be considered broad but the four questions subsequently posed add more specificity and focus. A further point to consider is that the question or objectives should be sufficiently narrow to make the review feasible. A feasible review is one where it is possible for all related studies to be identified. If the topic is too broad it may render it impossible to manage in terms of the numbers of studies that would have to be included.

It is fundamental that the research question and/or objectives are clearly focused. Some reviews frame the questions in terms of population, interventions, comparators, outcomes and study design (PICOS). What this means is that the review question includes reference to each of these elements. It is worth noting, however, that not all elements will always be relevant. For example, some review questions will not indicate the type of study design to be included (CRD, 2009). In addition, PICOS is normally used for reviews related to therapeutic interventions. Where qualitative studies are reviewed the acronym PEO (population, exposure, outcomes) can be used (Bettany-Saltikov, 2012). Box 3.1 outlines how these were included in an update of a Cochrane review to determine the effectiveness of planning the discharge of patients from hospital to home.

Population

In formulating a good question, the review team specifies the characteristics of the population or participants to be included. This incorporates outlining any inclusion or exclusion criteria in terms of age, gender, educational status or the presence of a particular disease or condition. The inclusion or exclusion of any of these factors is determined primarily by the topic of interest but should be broad enough to ensure that a range of studies are included. In the example cited in Box 3.1 the reviewers included all 'patients in hospital'.

Intervention/Comparators

Detail regarding the interventions to be included in the review should be specified also. These may include factors such as the type of intervention, where the intervention is delivered and the person administering the intervention. For example, in the review outlined in Box 3.1, while the intervention was broadly classed as 'structured discharge planning' the reviewers subsequently detailed specific criteria that delineated what they meant by 'structured' in the PICOS elements.

Similarly, if comparisons are to be included these should be described. In the example cited, the reviewers indicated that 'standard care with no structured discharge plan' constituted the comparator. Although it could be argued that the term 'standard care' was not specific enough, the essential delimiter for this review was the absence of an individualised and structured discharge plan. However, in other instances, defining terms is important in terms of being able to compare the findings of various studies. For instance, in a review undertaken by Spilsbury et al. (2011), the review question included reference to 'quality of care'. Given the complex nature of this concept it was fundamental that the reviewers specified clearly what they understood by this term.

Whiting (2009) highlighted that there are different types of comparisons and it is critical to specify which type will be examined so that the appropriate studies are sourced. For example, she outlines that the reviewer could focus on studies that compare one type of intervention with none at all (as in the cited example). Another possibility is to include studies where the focus is on identifying whether one form of intervention is preferable to another.

Outcomes

In the review question the reference to an outcome is usually stated in general terms related to the effectiveness of the intervention and might include statements such as 'assess the effects', 'determine the clinical effectiveness' or 'assess the clinical effectiveness'. The review team subsequently determine the types of outcome measures to be included. Higgins and Green (2008) state that outcomes can be related to a number of factors including mortality, clinical events, patient-reported outcomes, adverse effects, burden on patients and carers, and economic factors.

The outcomes in the discharge planning example in Box 3.1 were linked directly to the objective and questions for the review. For example, length of stay, readmission rate, complication rate and place of discharge were seen as factors that could determine if discharge planning improved the appropriate use of acute care in hospital while mortality rate, patient health status, patient and carer satisfaction, and psychological health of the patient and caregivers could establish if discharge planning improved or (at least) had no adverse effect on patient outcome.

Study Design

As indicated previously, review questions and objectives do not always include the type of studies to be included. However, they may be specified in the PICOS elements and developed in more detail in the remainder of the protocol. There are several factors that must be taken into consideration when deciding the type of study design to be included in the review. Essentially, the review question should direct the type of studies to be included. As indicated in Chapter 2, the logic of systematic reviews has been extended to incorporate a greater variety of research questions with the result that a broader range of evidence is needed to answer those questions.

For example, in systematic reviews of interventions, RCTs are the preferred type of study design for inclusion as they are seen to produce the most reliable and valid results. This is because the RCT study design has the most robust procedures for reducing susceptibility to bias. However, it may be that RCTs related to the topic area do not exist or are limited in number and, in these instances, quasi-experimental or observational studies that are not at the level of RCTs may be included (CRD, 2009). What is important though is that reviewers do not attempt to 'pool' the data from these different study designs because it makes comparison difficult and has implications for the validity of the findings.

There has been some discussion among the systematic review community about the contribution data from qualitative research can make to reviews of effectiveness (CRD, 2009; EPPI, 2010). This follows the recognition that although RCTs and quasi-experimental approaches may determine the most effective intervention, there are other factors that impact on its implementation, such as the experiences of people receiving it (CRD, 2009). Three options are suggested by CRD (2009: 222) for how qualitative evidence can be included in or alongside quantitative effectiveness reviews. Briefly these are: using the evidence from qualitative studies in the discussion of the quantitative synthesis; using the qualitative evidence to interpret the quantitative synthesis; or using a formal system combining the evidence from qualitative and quantitative studies. If qualitative evidence is to be included in or alongside an effectiveness review, it is important to outline in the protocol how this will be done.

To date, most systematic reviews incorporating qualitative evidence have been undertaken separately and many address questions that are not related directly to effectiveness. For instance, review topics or questions that are concerned with people's experiences could incorporate designs such as descriptive survey or qualitative research studies. For example, Brunton et al.'s (2011) research synthesis of women's experiences of having their first child ultimately selected studies that focused on open-ended qualitative approaches because they were more in keeping with the aims of the review.

A final point about study designs is that reviewers may not be in a position in the initial stages to determine which study designs are to be included and, therefore, they may not appear in the PICOS elements.

Box 3.1   PICOS Elements of a Systematic Review: Discharge Planning from Hospital to Home (Shepperd et al., 2010)

Objective of the review

To determine the effectiveness of planning the discharge of patients from hospital to home.

Questions

1 Does discharge planning improve the appropriate use of acute care?
2 Does discharge planning improve or (at least) have no adverse effect on patient outcome?
3 Does discharge planning reduce overall costs of health care?

Population (Participants)

The studies to be included in the review included all hospital inpatients (acute, rehabilitation or community) irrespective of age, gender or condition.

Intervention – Structured Discharge Planning

Studies were included if the structured discharge plans included:

- pre-admission assessment (where possible).
- case finding on admission.
- inpatient assessment and preparation of a discharge plan based on an individual patient's need.
- implementation of the discharge plan.
- monitoring.

Comparators

The control group had to receive standard care with no structured discharge planning.

Outcomes

- Length of stay in hospital.
- Readmission rate to hospital.
- Complication rate.
- Place of discharge.
- Mortality rate.
- Patient-health status.
- Patient satisfaction.
- Carer satisfaction.
- Psychological health of patient.
- Psychological health of caregivers.
- Cost of discharge planning to the hospital and to the community.
- The use of medication for trials evaluating a pharmacy discharge plan.

Study Design

Randomised controlled trials that compared an individualised discharge plan with routine discharge care that was not tailored to the individual patient.

Identifying Studies for Inclusion

The first step in identifying studies for inclusion in the review is detailing the criteria by which they will be included or excluded. In essence, these criteria constitute the search strategy and define the parameters of the review. They include defining search terms, describing how the literature is searched and outlining delimiters such as publication types, timelines and language. They are in addition to any criteria that have been identified already in the PICOS or PEO elements. The inclusion and exclusion criteria are normally determined in the planning stage of the review so as to reduce the potential for bias. This is based on the view that if decisions are made in advance (a priori) then the reviewers are not influenced or swayed by the findings of individual studies. However, there are times when a more emergent process may be adopted and, whilst this may be seen as contrary to the systematic review process, the key factor is that the reviewers adhere to the principles of being transparent and explicit (Marshall et al., 2011).

Decisions regarding inclusion or exclusion criteria must be justified as they are likely to have implications for the overall validity of the findings. For example, if a reviewer chooses to source publications in English only, important evidence may be missed, which will have implications for the overall outcome of the review. However, factors such as time and resources may limit the reviewers' ability to source all studies related to the topic. For instance, retrieving published or even unpublished research in another language may be time consuming and there may be the added cost of translating that work. The important point is that these are recognised as possible limitations and will impact on how, for example, the findings can be generalised. Areas that are commonly addressed in systematic reviews in respect of inclusion or exclusion criteria are outlined in Box 3.2. Further detail on each of these can be found in Chapter 4.

Box 3.2   Inclusion/Exclusion Criteria

Search Terms

Specification of the key terms.

Identifying Sources of Literature

- Electronic databases.
- Manual/handsearching.
- Bibliography and references lists.
- Grey literature.

Publication Type

- Journals.
- Books or book chapters.
- Reports.
- Theses (published/unpublished).

- Conference abstracts.
- Conference papers.
- Interim reports.
- Unpublished work.
- Consulting with experts in the field.

Language Delimiters

Inclusions/exclusions by virtue of the language of publication.

Timelines

Deciding on time limits for the review.

When reviewers are making decisions about their search strategy there are a number of factors that should be kept in mind. In respect of search terms, for example, Marshall et al. (2011) report how terminology, such as 'language', 'communication' and 'speech', commonly used in speech and language therapy has wider application in lay contexts and other disciplines. In instances such as these there is potential for large amounts of irrelevant literature to be generated and considerable skill is needed to manage this. In reality, very few searches are straightforward and reviewers will often include or seek the services of a librarian because of their professional expertise in searching and retrieval.

Even though electronic databases have eased the process of searching the literature, no single database records all healthcare publications. Moreover, not all published research is indexed in the main databases, thus making it more difficult to retrieve. In addition, it should be remembered that not all research is published in journals. Therefore, there is a need to search widely and include a range of sources such as those outlined in Box 3.2.

There are also issues with publication and language bias that should be kept in mind. For example, publications that have positive results are published more frequently than those with negative results (Whiting, 2009). Also, language bias refers to the tendency for authors to seek publication in English language journals if the results are positive or statistically significant (Bettany-Saltikov, 2012).

Catling-Paull et al. (2011: 1647–8) used the search strategy outlined below in their systematic review of 'clinical interventions that increase the uptake and success of vaginal birth after caesarean section'. Examine the search strategy and assess it for completeness or any possible biases.

Keywords used

'Intervention' and 'Pregnancy Outcome' with 'Vaginal Birth After C(a)esarean/Caesarian', 'VBAC', 'Trial of Labo(u)r', C(a)esarean/Caesarian Section' and 'C(a)esarean/Caesarian Section, repeat'.

ACTIVITY 3.1

(Continued)

(Continued)

Unrestricted search

- CDSR (Cochrane Database of Systematic Reviews).
- CINAHL (Cumulative Index to Nursing & Allied Health).
- Ovid MEDLINE(R).
- MIDIRS (Maternity and Infant Care).
- PsycINFO was undertaken to determine any studies that evaluated an intervention for vaginal birth after caesarean section (VBAC).
- Government health websites and obstetric and midwifery professional organisation websites.
- Reference lists of relevant articles, including any guidelines and reviews.

Included

- Studies written in English that evaluated an intervention for increasing either the uptake of and/or the success of VBAC.
- Studies that involved a comparison group (randomised controlled trials, cohort studies, case control studies and before-and-after studies); and published up to December 2008.

Excluded

- Studies that did not report VBAC uptake or success rates were excluded.
- Only primary sources were considered appropriate for this review. Systematic reviews were used to source further publications but were excluded as they were not primary sources.

Study Selection

Following retrieval of the literature, the reviewers detail how studies were selected for inclusion. Study selection is normally done in two stages, which involves an initial screening followed by screening of the full papers. The initial screening includes judging the titles and/or abstracts of the studies against the inclusion criteria. Those that do not match the criteria are rejected immediately. Where there is some doubt, it is better to access the full paper rather than exclude too early. The second stage involves detailed screening of the full papers against the inclusion criteria. It is important that more than one person considers the eligibility of a study for inclusion. This will reduce the risk of relevant papers being discarded inadvertently. It may be helpful to construct a flow chart of how studies were selected (see Figure 3.1).

Throughout the searching and retrieval of literature, it is fundamental that all decisions are carefully recorded and, in particular, when studies are excluded. It is also important to 'manage' the retrieved literature, and there are many bibliographic software packages available for that purpose.

In some systematic reviews, a descriptive mapping exercise may be undertaken whereby an overview of the research literature available on a given topic is presented (EPPI, 2010). This may be done as part of a two-stage review where the original topic is very broad. Through descriptive mapping, the reviewers develop a clearer picture of the subject following which they narrow the focus or refine the original review question. In other instances, where what are deemed to be an unmanageable

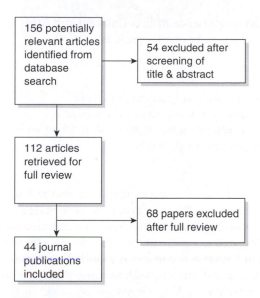

Figure 3.1   Example of Flowchart from Database Search

number of references are retrieved and if the review team does not have the capacity or resources to conduct an in-depth review of all the retrieved material, the scope of the review is narrowed. It may also be that narrowing or refining the topic will ultimately have more useful outcomes for end-users (EPPI, 2010).

Quality Assessment

The next step in the process of undertaking a systematic review is to assess the quality of the studies that are included. In all literature reviews, there is an expectation that reviewers make some judgement about the quality of the work. However, how well and the extent to which it is done is largely dependent on the reviewers and their skills. In a systematic review, it is a key requirement of the process because the strength of the findings or conclusions of the review are dependent on the quality of the original studies included.

In systematic reviews where the included studies are quantitative, the criteria for judging quality are largely concerned with determining if sufficiently robust steps were taken to reduce methodological bias in the design, conduct and analysis of the study. What this means, in essence, is that various aspects of the primary studies must be examined to determine the 'truthfulness' or 'believability' of the original findings. It also enables the reviewers to judge whether variations between the results of one study and another can be explained by differences in quality.

While the emphasis will vary depending on the focus and type of review being undertaken, the criteria for judging studies that fall under the umbrella of quantitative designs generally include:

- deciding if the chosen research design was appropriate for answering the research question or aim.

- identifying the risk or presence of bias (internal validity).
- other issues related to study quality such as:

  o considering the reliability and validity of the measuring tool or instrument used.
  o statistical issues around sampling and analysis.
  o the quality of reporting of aspects of the study.
  o assessing if the intervention has been used appropriately.
  o generalisability (external validity).
  (CRD, 2009: 33)

Although there is a wide range of instruments available to critically appraise studies, more recently a number of specific tools have been developed for research design. This is important because systematic reviews involving 'quantitative' studies tend to focus on one or very similar research designs. For example, the review may only include RCTs. Therefore, rather than having a broad-based tool that appraises 'quantitative' studies in general, design-specific instruments, such as those developed as part of the Critical Appraisal Skills Programme (CASP) (www.sph.nhs.uk), focus on methodological questions that have relevance and are explicit to the design of the study being assessed.

However, in systematic reviews that incorporate qualitative studies it is likely that more than one type of research design will be included, and appraisal of quality must accommodate this. Yet, there is little consensus among qualitative researchers about the question of quality. Despite the number of frameworks that have been developed for assessing quality, in qualitative research debates continue about their appropriateness. Some consider that it is not possible to develop a single tool that addresses all qualitative research given the diverse philosophical, theoretical and methodological positions that exist.

Nonetheless, quality assessment is a fundamental part of the process and it is important that reviewers determine how the research evidence that is to be used is both trustworthy and relevant. EPPI (2010) provide some useful guidelines in this respect. They indicate that in the first instance reviewers should evaluate the methodological quality of the studies independently of the review question. In doing so they make a judgement as to whether or not the study meets the acknowledged standards for the chosen research design. In this way, the trustworthiness of the study is determined. This is similar to what you would do in any literature review and a tool such as that outlined in Chapter 6 might be applicable.

Subsequently, the reviewers would make a judgement about the study's relevance in terms of answering the review question. EPPI (2010) have identified two such aspects as 'methodological relevance' and 'topic relevance'. Methodological relevance is concerned with deciding if the study design or methodology used answers the review question or contributes to the review's conclusions. For example, in Brunton et al.'s (2011) research synthesis of women's views of the experience of first-time motherhood, 'quantitative' designs that used rating scales or measurement instruments to collect data were ultimately excluded as it was concluded that they did not permit women to talk about their 'experiences' outside the preset tools.

The second issue of topic relevance is concerned with assessing variations in the focus of the topic, the population used or the context in which it was used. If we use Brunton et al.'s (2011) synthesis again as an example, on the advice of their advisory group that consisted of researchers, practitioners and policy customers they confined the review to UK-based studies because of their relevance and potential benefit for most end-users. As part of the appraisal of studies, reviewers may choose to develop a scoring system for each criterion in the quality assessment. The scores are aggregated and the studies are classed, usually, as being of a high, medium or low quality.

Important aspects of undertaking the quality assessment will be deciding what checklist, quality criteria and/or scoring system will be used. Decisions about the impact of the scoring of studies should be clear. For example, it may be that studies that are considered of a medium or low quality may not be excluded but that a system is developed to 'weight' the evidence. What this means is that studies that are of good quality and are larger in terms of their size might be given more 'weight'. Therefore, when reading a systematic review you should be able to discern how the reviewers have done this.

In addition, the assessment is usually undertaken independently by more than one person. Therefore, it is important to decide how many people will be involved, how decisions regarding the final inclusion and/or exclusion of studies will be made and how disagreements are resolved. The advisory group or panel can also advise in terms of ensuring that the quality assessment has been undertaken appropriately. If a systematic review is being undertaken as a postgraduate study, then the role of the supervisor in assisting with and reviewing the quality assessment process is central.

Data Extraction

Data extraction is the means by which the information is taken from the studies included in the review. It is known at this point of the review that all selected studies are relevant to the research question and have met the inclusion criteria. Now the reviewers return to each study and extract the information that will answer the question. Normally, a data extraction form is developed and utilised to record the information. However, these are not standardised and it is important that the criteria are tailored to the individual review. Nonetheless, where PICO or PEO criteria have been used data are extracted according to the elements identified therein. The Cochrane Handbook (Higgins and Green, 2008), the CRD's (2009) guidance for systematic reviews and EPPI's (2010) methods for conducting systematic reviews all provide guidance for what should be included in data extraction forms for various types of systematic review.

As with quality assessment, more than one person may perform the data extraction in order to reduce bias and enhance the reliability of the process and strategies. However, there is an inherent risk that those extracting the data may not do so consistently. Therefore, it is important to pilot the data extraction form on a sample of the included studies to make certain that the reviewers are interpreting in a consistent way but also to ensure the tool itself is capturing the pertinent data (CRD, 2009).

Data Synthesis

Discussion of data synthesis here is limited to an outline as further detail on the process is presented in Chapter 7. When all the data have been extracted, the information is synthesised, which at its simplest means pulling together all the evidence. Like most stages of a systematic review how this is done depends on the purpose of the review. However, it should begin with a descriptive summary and presentation of the findings. At the very least this should include a collation of information about each study, which is then presented in a grid or table. (See Boxes 3.3 and 3.4 for how this might be done.) Reviewers may also use individual illustrations, figures or tables that aid understanding. Most reviews will contain a descriptive or narrative summary or synthesis to support the tabular and graphic illustrations.

Box 3.3   Example of a Summary Table

Title	Author/ Year	Full reference	Methods	Participants	Interventions	Outcomes	Risk of bias

Box 3.4   Example of a Summary Table

Title	Author/Year	Full reference	Aims	Method	Population	Quality rating

Data synthesis has been likened to data analysis (Hamer and Collinson, 2005). As indicated above, how the analysis is conducted depends on the purpose of the review and the type of studies that have been included in it. For example, if a review included only RCTs then a statistical analysis known as meta-analysis may be undertaken whereby the data from the included studies is pooled and re-analysed as one large data set with the purpose of calculating a 'single summary statistic' or 'effect measure' (Booth et al., 2010: 294). This enables meaningful conclusions to be drawn across studies because combining the results increases the chance of detecting that a 'real' effect is statistically significant (CRD, 2009).

However, meta-analysis is not always possible or even desired. For example, as indicated in Chapter 2, not all healthcare questions can be answered by RCTs. Moreover, where non-randomised studies using a range of research designs have been included in the review then meta-analysis is not recommended (CRD, 2009). Therefore, where statistical analysis is not undertaken, a narrative synthesis is conducted.

Studies that are not suitable for meta-analysis may include experimental and non-experimental studies that are too heterogeneous (diverse) or have used a range of different research designs. Traditionally, however, there have been difficulties associated with narrative synthesis in that there is no clear guidance for establishing the credibility or trustworthiness of the adopted approaches. Popay et al. (2006) identified a general framework that suggests a narrative synthesis should include four elements: developing a theory of how the intervention works, why and for whom; developing a preliminary synthesis of the findings; exploring relationships within and across the studies; and assessing if the synthesis is robust.

Barnett-Page and Thomas (2009) state that narrative synthesis is a term that is used more frequently when referring to synthesis of quantitative research. Within the qualitative research community a number of methods and terms have emerged to describe the various means for synthesising qualitative research. This proliferation of terms and methods and the surrounding debates can be confusing for the reader and perhaps for those who are considering undertaking a systematic review of qualitative research and want to choose the best method. However, whilst an absolute consensus does not exist, the term meta-synthesis has emerged as one that encompasses various approaches to synthesising qualitative research studies (Paterson et al., 2009). Some of these methods include but are not limited to meta-ethnography, meta-study, meta-narrative, meta-summary, thematic synthesis, critical interpretive synthesis and grounded theory. To date, meta-ethnography is the most commonly used method. A useful summary of the some of these methods is provided by Ring et al. (2010).

Whilst there are variations in how the synthesis is conducted, most methods are concerned with interpretation, that is, deconstructing the research findings from each study, discovering key features and combining them again in a transformed whole. The outcome then is a new interpretation that is greater than the sum of the individual studies (Flemming, 2007; Finlayson and Dixon, 2008). These new insights are often represented as concepts or theories. Lindahl and Lindblad's (2011) meta-synthesis of 'family member's experiences of everyday life when a child is dependent on a ventilator' is a useful example of the process. Meta-summary differs as a method of synthesising qualitative data as it has been described as 'aggregative', that is, the results are assembled, pooled and summarised rather than being interpreted (Finfgeld-Connett, 2010).

Undertaking a meta-synthesis using whichever method is a complex and challenging endeavour, not least in respect of the analysis phase. Not only is the process time consuming but it is also fraught with unresolved issues. For example, debate continues about combining studies that are philosophically, theoretically and methodologically diverse. Some consider that this should not be done while others believe that it is synthesising the findings that is the main focus (Bondas and Hall, 2007). In addition, the reviewer may be faced with the difficulty of combining studies that have different populations and/or contradictory or conflicting findings. Nonetheless, a key factor is that like the synthesis of quantitative data, it is important that whatever method is chosen it is conducted rigorously and is transparent to the reader.

Presentation and Discussion of Results

As with all research, once the analysis (synthesis) stage has been completed the reviewers turn their attention to presenting and discussing the results of the review. While the manner in which the results are presented varies, the purpose of the discussion is to facilitate interpretation of the findings of the review. Essentially, the discussion should include the analysis of the findings, the meaning of the findings and the strengths and weaknesses of the review.

Some reviewers prefer to integrate the presentation of findings with a discussion of them while others present them separately. Either way, it is important that the discussion reviews the findings in light of the original aim and objectives and the relevant theoretical and background literature (Bettany-Saltikov, 2012). This should involve comparing and contrasting the results with the work of others in the field and making interpretations or judgements as to their implications, say for practice or policy. The discussion may also address theoretical considerations, such as making a claim for a new conceptualisation of a phenomenon. For example, Beck's (2002) meta-synthesis of 18 qualitative studies on post-partum depression yielded four overarching themes of 'pervasive loss', 'incongruity between expectations and reality of motherhood', 'making gains' and 'spiralling downward' that had subsumed within them metaphors and concepts that had been identified in each study. This synthesis of the findings of all the available studies offered a new conceptualisation of post-partum depression that could be the basis for the development of theory, which in turn would have implications for practice and research.

The discussion should include, where applicable, a commentary on aspects of the studies included in the review, such as their ethical integrity or their quality and whether they had an influence on the findings. Clear recommendations for professional practice, theoretical development and further research/enquiry should be presented also. Particular attention should be given to these recommendations, as they are often the key area of interest to practitioners, policy makers and consumers of services. Just as in any research, it is important to include remarks on the methodological limitations of the review but also to present the strengths, difficulties and/or challenges that were encountered throughout.

How the report is written will vary depending on whether the review was conducted for a commissioning body, as an academic piece of work such as a dissertation, or for a journal article. Some commissioning bodies, libraries and journals have their own recommendations for how results of systematic reviews are presented. In addition, guidelines such as those found on the EQUATOR network (Enhancing the Quality and Transparency of Health Research) (www.equator-network.org) provides guidance for authors on reporting and publishing so that the quality of their work is enhanced. Currently, for systematic reviews this is restricted to the Preferred Reporting Items for Systematic Reviews and Meta-Analyses (PRISMA) (Moher et al., 2009) and the Meta-analysis Of Observational Studies in Epidemiology (MOOSE) (Stroup et al., 2000). However, other organisations such as the Cochrane collaboration, CRD and EPPI all provide guidelines on reporting.

Dissemination of Review Findings

The final and vital part of a systematic review is dissemination of the findings, which is essential to ensuring the message reaches its intended audience be they practitioners, end-users, policy makers, organisations or commissioners of research. Inherent in this is the need to recognise that dissemination is an active process that should have been planned at the protocol stage. It is also important that the manner in which the message is conveyed is understood by the recipients. This may mean that the results of the review may be disseminated more widely and through different media than the traditional academic journals or conferences (CRD, 2009).

Summary

This chapter has provided an overview of the process of undertaking a systematic review. Systematic reviews were identified as research studies that follow an explicit and transparent methodology whereby evidence from previously conducted primary studies is re-analysed and synthesised. The steps involved in undertaking a systematic review were presented. Although systematic reviews were traditionally associated with reviews of effectiveness of interventions, this chapter has outlined how the method has been evolving, and the types of questions being addressed and the methods for synthesising the evidence from a wide range of study designs have expanded. Whilst this chapter largely follows the standard protocol, variations – particularly in the synthesis methods – have been presented to demonstrate how the process has advanced in recent years. Undertaking a systematic review is a complex endeavour but you should now have some insight into the method and be able to distinguish the range of purposes for which such a review might be undertaken.

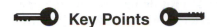 **Key Points**

- A systematic review is a research study that follows an explicit and transparent methodology to re-analyse and synthesise evidence from previously conducted primary studies.
- Systematic reviews were developed originally to review effectiveness of interventions using RCTs and quasi-experimental approaches. However, their use is continually expanding and now includes studies, such as qualitative research, that are not related directly to effectiveness.
- Regardless of the type of studies that are being reviewed, a review protocol (plan) must be prepared prior to undertaking any systematic review. The protocol details the purpose of the review; the research question and objectives; the search strategy; the plan for analysis, interpretation and presentation of the data; and how the results will be disseminated.
- A systematic review begins with the development of a research question that may be framed using PICOS or PEO elements.
- Study design, identification of studies for inclusion in the review, selection of studies, quality assessment, data extraction, data synthesis, presentation and discussion of results, and dissemination constitute the main features of a systematic review although there are variations, particularly in respect of how data is synthesised.

4

Selecting a Review Topic and Searching the Literature

Introduction

As stated in Chapter 1, there are a number of reasons for undertaking a literature review. Whatever the reason for doing a review, the first next step is always identifying the topic to be reviewed or researched. The review, whether it is a work in its own right or part of a larger study, needs careful consideration. A literature review takes time to complete and can be demanding. It is therefore worthwhile identifying a topic that will hold your interest throughout. If the literature review is an academic assignment it is important to read the accompanying guidelines as there may be considerations, such as the topic being linked to a specialist area or subject, for example drug dependence, a time frame in which the review must be completed, or a word limit. All these will influence, in one way or another, your choice of topic. Undertaking a review that is linked to a specialist subject obviously limits the topics that can be selected. In academic assignments time frames can entail a penalty if the work is not completed by the due date. This can limit the type of literature that you may be able to access, for example inter-library loans, and therefore the choice of topic. Another difficulty linked to this is that novice reviewers often underestimate the time it takes to do a review, and while searching and gathering the literature is an important aspect of a literature review they are only a part of what is required. Similarly, word limits usually have consequences if a limit is not met or is exceeded; therefore the topic needs to have the depth to meet the word count but not be so vast that it can only be superficially presented. Thus, a word limit can force you to be concise within the review, and therefore it is essential to have a clear aim when you are selecting the topic of interest.

☑ **Learning Outcomes** ☑

By the end of this chapter you should be able to:

- identify and refine a topic of interest.
- recognise sources and types of literature.
- develop a search strategy.
- Identify keywords and phrases.
- limit or expand a search.

Identifying a Research Topic/Problem

Identifying and selecting a topic to review is probably the most important aspect of a literature review or a research study. It is the first step in undertaking a literature review and, if poorly conceived, can often leave you feeling overwhelmed and perhaps considering abandoning the whole process. Alternatively, an interesting, manageable problem can be the driving force that encourages you to ask questions, seek answers and stay motivated. Finding a manageable topic can be a difficult task for both students and novice reviewers alike, and so it is important to spend time carefully considering the topic before undertaking a literature review. Topics can be identified from a number of sources, some of which are displayed in Box 4.1. Other topic sources are equally valid, and it is often a combination of sources that helps to formulate a research question.

Box 4.1   Topic Sources

Professional/Clinical Practice

Issues and problems commonly encountered in clinical practice can be the source of an idea for a literature review. As these problems are professional in nature they tend to arouse greater interest and be more relevant to the reviewer as the outcomes can inform practice.

Reading the Literature

Research and opinion articles can be a good starting point in identifying a topic of interest. Research recommendations often identify areas for further review and study, and comments from journal articles can stimulate discussions and debates leading to a review of the literature on the topic.

Quality Assurance

Ensuring and improving quality of care is an expectation of all healthcare professionals. Topics can include identifying ways of improving care, patients' perceptions of care, or

(Continued)

(Continued)

reviewing methods of measuring quality to identify the most appropriate method for a particular clinical environment.

Contemporary Issues

These can include current social and cultural issues that can be identified through the media or through publications from government or other organisations. Problems that might be identified include hospital overcrowding or equality of access to health or social services.

(Adapted from Polit and Beck, 2012)

Clinical practice is one of the most favoured sources of topics for both reviews and research studies. Topics from practice have the benefit of being of interest and can also help you to develop professionally. Practice-based topics can arise out of issues or incidents that occur in the clinical area or other areas of professional practice and may stimulate questions such as 'Is there an alternative way of managing this?' or 'Why is the outcome different for this patient?'

Whatever the topic, it is important that you ascertain clearly what is of interest, as it may not be practical to attempt a review without a precise understanding of what is being investigated. It can be useful to brainstorm with friends and colleagues to help you define and refine the problem. It is also worthwhile discussing your ideas with clinical and subject specialists who can often offer alternative perspectives on the topic.

Refining the Research Topic

Refining the research topic can sometimes be like the chicken and egg scenario. The purpose of refining the topic is to enable a reasonably focused review of the literature to be undertaken, yet in order to get a greater insight into the topic and perhaps identify specifically the area of interest, knowledge of the literature is required. A review topic frequently starts out as a broad area of interest, such as pain. While this may be a useful starting point – 'I am interested in something to do with pain', pain is such a broad topic in itself that the amount of literature associated with it will be so vast as to leave the review impractical. A search on one database for pain led to 262,287 hits and numerous sub-categories (see Box 4.2). A quick search such as this can be useful as it can identify these sub-categories, which can be helpful in refining the topic and can also indicate how much literature is available on the topic. The latter is particularly important if the review is an academic assignment. Assignments often have tight deadlines so it is a good idea to identify a topic with sufficient literature (Timmins and McCabe, 2005) as it can make completion of the review and submission by the due date easier. Gould (2008) recommends a preliminary search to identify what has been studied in relation to the topic. Some aspects of the topic may have attracted a lot of interest, which in turn can lead to a lot of hits in relation to this area. Other aspects may have attracted a more moderate interest, which may be more appropriate to the length of the review and the time frame it has to be completed within.

Box 4.2   Sub-categories for Pain

- Pain and middle age.
- Pain and pain measurement.
- Pain management.
- Pain and pain management.
- Pain assessment.
- Pain and analgesics.
- Pain and chronic disease.
- Pain and treatment outcomes.
- Pain and patients.
- Muscle pain.
- Analgesics.

Returning to pain as the topic of interest, it is clear that this needs to be refined to make it more specific and so more manageable. It is worth considering what it is about pain that is of interest. Is there a specific element, such as pain management or post-operative pain that has caught your attention? Recognising what precisely is of interest and why can go a long way to refining the topic of interest.

Identifying Literature Sources

Once the topic of interest has been refined and a research problem or purpose has been identified, the next step is to start considering the literature. Literature is usually considered as being published written material, but in some instances material that is unpublished or comes from an alternative media source, such as television or radio, may be utilised. The literature to be used within a review should be gathered in an organised manner and should be appropriate and related to the research question or topic of interest. A systematic approach to gathering the literature is usually expected in an academic review, and while this does not imply a 'systematic review', some of the principles of this type of review are required. These include:

- identifying a well-defined aim or purpose for your review at the outset, so it is clear to the reader what is being investigated.
- identifying how the data was categorised and selected for the review – this includes listing the databases and search engines used, other searches undertaken, the key words or search terms used and how the search was limited.

Having a clearly defined aim at this point is important because the more specific you can be when searching the literature, the greater the likelihood that the material identified will be relevant to, and reflect the purpose of, the review. The more relevant the identified material is the more probable that the review will be focused on the area of interest. Again this is important as there is an expectation of depth of reading and discussion around the area of interest, and this can be difficult to achieve where there is a lack of focus. A clearly defined aim also allows for easier recognition of the themes or concepts that underpin this idea or hypothesis, and this can be useful in identifying the most appropriate databases or literature sources as well as the most suitable keywords.

Categorising the Literature

It is important to know what sort of literature best suits the review being undertaken and the research question being asked. Literature can be classified under a number of different headings, and while there may be an overlap in what types of literature are used within a review, the focus of the review or research question will determine which type of literature will be most useful. Literature is categorised by how it presents knowledge (Price, 2009) and includes research, theoretical, philosophical, experiential/practice and policy literature.

Research literature, as its name suggests, comprises literature from research studies, including both quantitative and qualitative studies, as well as results from systematic literature reviews, and meta-analysis and meta-synthesis studies. This type of literature is important if the purpose of the review is to explore a topic to discover facts or principles (Price, 2009).

Theoretical literature differs from research in that it suggests reasons to explain phenomena or predict responses in particular situations, such as how an individual may respond to grief or loss (Kübler-Ross, 1969). Theories are there to be tested so this type of literature is not totally separate from research in that theories often inform, support or are tested as part of a research study and can therefore be important literature sources.

Philosophical literature deals with attitudes and beliefs in relation to concepts such as health, illness and caring (Price, 2009). It also includes ethical and moral considerations in relation to issues such as withholding treatment or the right to die.

Experiential/practice literature is usually written by individuals with an expertise within an area and who wish to share their experiences with others in the field. This literature can be presented in the form of case studies (Price, 2009), as discussion papers or other forms of expert opinion (Aveyard, 2010).

Policy literature includes local, national and international guidelines and policies that advocate best practice. Policies and guidelines are usually evidence based when developed, but need to be updated on a regular basis. This type of literature can again be useful in setting a context for a review or highlighting a standard that should be achieved. However, it is worth mentioning again that the guidelines or policies you are referring to should be the most recent and up to date.

Sourcing the Literature

Literature for a review can be obtained from a number of sources. While it may be acceptable for small academic literature reviews to be confined to a number of professional databases, for larger and more in-depth reviews multiple sources of literature are recommended. Greenhalgh and Peacock (2005) advocate using multiple approaches to searching the literature and not being confined solely to one form of search. Important publications can be missed because, for example, they are poorly indexed. Poor indexing can occur for a number of reasons (Evans, 2002; Montori et al., 2005). Among these are the use of amusing or entertaining titles (Hawker et al., 2002), and this can be particularly the case in qualitative studies. It is therefore important, for a systematic search, to use as many search methods and sources as possible. A number of literature sources are included in Box 4.3.

Box 4.3   Sources of Literature

- Electronic databases and Internet search engines.
- Catalogues.
- Grey literature – conference proceedings, unpublished literature (PhD or Masters studies).
- Textbooks and dictionaries.
- Manual searches.

Database and Internet Searches

Literature searches are now mainly undertaken online. In fact, most libraries have now moved to online journals as this allows multiple individuals access at the same time, and reduces storage problems and the difficulties of replacing journals that have gone astray. Databases and search engines are the major sources of information and literature for reviewers and researchers. Databases are the most common way to search for professional literature. Databases are organised collections of literature stored in an electronic format. The collections are usually derived from journals, books, dissertations, reviews and conference proceedings, and include full text, abstracts and references of works selected. While some databases can be accessed for free, a membership subscription is normally required; universities, colleges and organisations such as hospitals, however, will usually have institutional subscriptions to one or more databases and provide access to staff and students associated with that institution. Some databases that may be of interest are shown in Table 4.1.

Search engines are computer programs that can be used to search the Internet for information specified by the searcher. The information presented by a search engine is in the form of 'a web page' that can then offer specific information or redirect the searcher to other sites. Because different search engines, such as Bing, Dogpile, Google, Google Scholar and Yahoo, use their own unique software programs to trawl the Internet using the same search terms on different search engines can sometimes yield different results. It is therefore worthwhile using a variety of search engines.

Search engines can be useful tools when searching for documents and reports from government agencies, professional bodies, voluntary and professional agencies and self-help groups. They can also be used to access databases and other useful sites. However, Ely and Scott (2007) offer a word of warning regarding using the Internet

Table 4.1   Nursing, Health and Social Care Related Databases

Database	Main Content	Access
Allied and Complementary Medicine Database (AMED)	Journals related to allied health literature, complementary medicine and palliative care.	Subscription required
British Nursing Index (BNI)	Nursing journals, mainly of UK origin.	Subscription required
Centre for Reviews and Dissemination (CRD)	Systematic reviews and meta-analysis for evidence-based medicine.	Free access
Cochrane Library	Database of systematic reviews.	Free access (UK and Ireland)
Cumulative Index to Nursing and Allied Health Literature (CINAHL)	Journals related to nursing and allied health issues.	Subscription required
Joanna Briggs Institute	Evidence-based research relating to nursing and allied health care.	Subscription required
MEDLINE/PubMed	Journals related to life sciences, particularly biomedicine. Free access to this database is available through PubMed.	Free access
Social Care Online	This site offers access to UK government documents and reports, and journal articles related to social care and social work.	Free access
Proquest Nursing and Allied Health Source	Covers journals related to nursing and allied health, including physical and occupational therapy, and rehabilitation.	Subscription required
PsycINFO	This database contains peer-reviewed journals related to mental health and the behavioural sciences.	Subscription required

as a source of information, stating that web pages can be posted by any individual and can include personal views and unsupported commentaries. Therefore, it is important to carefully check the reliability of the information offered on the Internet and only use recognised, trustworthy sites.

Catalogues

Before the advent of the Internet and databases, professional data was stored in catalogues or printed indices, which were available for searching in most university and college libraries. Depending on the type of review being undertaken it may be necessary to access these catalogues. However, this can be a time-consuming and therefore expensive search. Electronic cataloguing of articles in many databases is only available from 1982 (Rebar et al., 2011), and while MEDLINE includes articles back to the 1940s, literature before 1982 will generally have to be searched through the printed medium. Catalogues for databases were categorised by author and topic and updated annually; thus, you will have to search the selected databases one year at a time if using these in a review.

Grey Literature

The so-called 'grey literature' includes data from conference proceedings and unpublished works, such as Masters and PhD studies. This can be important information from the point of view of being comprehensive. However, at undergraduate and even at Masters level, the benefits have to be weighed against the cost in time to undertake the search, the cost financially if this literature has to be accessed through inter-library loan and whether is is a requirement of the course to include such data in the review. Universities and third-level institutions usually have repositories that will identify some of the grey literature that is generated by their own establishment, and some information can be accessed through the Internet, and the GreyNet (www. greynet.org) and the Index to Theses (www.these.com) databases. However, searching for grey literature can be time consuming, especially if the searcher is unclear about what exactly is being sought.

Textbooks and Dictionaries

Textbooks are another useful source of information, especially for background on your topic and literature for initial reading. University or college library catalogues are often a good place to start searching these. However, one issue with textbooks is that they quickly become dated as 12 months or more may elapse between a book having been written and appearing in a bookshop. Libraries also frequently hold a number of older editions of books, so textbooks should be read with caution when seeking up-to-date sources of information. Dictionaries and thesauruses can be helpful for defining terms and concepts, and can prove useful when you are attempting to identify keywords.

Manual Searches

Another source of literature can be gained through manual searches. Manual searches are done to supplement database and other forms of searches. There are a number of ways to undertake a manual search and the ones included here are by no means exclusive.

One easy form of manual searching is to review the reference lists in articles that you have selected in your search of the databases. This can be particularly useful with recently published articles as they are most likely to have reasonably up-to-date reference lists. Ridley (2008) calls this the snowball technique and adds that some databases may allow you to track articles to identify other works that have cited them. This can be particularly useful for identifying who has cited seminal works in your area of interest as more than likely those who cited the work will be of interest. Published literature reviews can be very useful if searching in this way. However, it is important to source the original works, the primary sources, rather than using the review to describe and/or critically review the identified works. This is because you have no means of authenticating the comments in the review without accessing the original article. Citing from a secondary source, that is an author who makes reference to a primary source, should only be done if the primary work is inaccessible to the reviewer.

As you become familiar with the literature in a particular area, you will frequently be able to identify a number of authors who write extensively in that area. In such a case an author search can help to identify other works written by that person in the particular field. This type of search is usually difficult to undertake before searching the databases unless an author is particularly associated with that subject.

Another kind of manual search is a trawl through research journals. This can be particularly useful if the topic of interest is related to a specialist area supported by one or more dedicated journals. This search may involve reviewing the content index for each issue of that journal to identify relevant articles.

Searching and Selecting the Literature

One of the first considerations, before undertaking a search, is to decide how you will record it. Good notes on how the search was undertaken – for example, the databases searched and the keywords used – will make writing up the methodology of the search much easier. The methodology should describe the search to the extent that another reviewer could undertake the same search and identify much the same works. It will probably never be the same result, as databases are continuously updated. However, the person replicating the review should be able, at least, to locate the same literature you did. An example of how a literature search might be documented can be seen in a review by Akerjordet and Severinsson (2007) who described their search in relation to emotional intelligence (EI)(Box 4.4).

Box 4.4   Example of Documenting a Literature Search

A search was made of the MEDLINE, CINAHL and PsycInfo databases for the 15-year period from January 1990 to March 2005 to provide an overview of the scientific developmental process of EI. A manual search of relevant journals and significant references, including theoretical articles related to the topic, was also conducted. The search words used were: EI, empirical research, methods, philosophical and reviews. The outcome of the search revealed 926 abstracts including several dissertations, mainly comprising quantitative research approaches, non-empirical articles, anecdotal reports, editorials, news, comments, as well as theoretical and empirical research articles.

The selection was confined to identify articles published during the last 10 years, since the search revealed that no empirical or philosophical articles were published before 1995, which meant that 915 of the original 926 abstracts were relevant. Secondly, only articles published in English and focusing on empirical and philosophical approaches were included, which reduced the number of articles for analysis to 224. Only one article had a philosophical approach. The final analysis included a total of 16 papers, which were examined in detail in relation to original empirical research.

(Akerjordet and Severinsson, 2007: 1405–6)

Modern approaches to literature searching make locating literature a lot easier. However, searching is a skill that has to be learned and developed and is one that can sometimes prove frustrating for novice searchers. Common complaints by novice searchers are that there is little or no literature that relates to their area of interest or that they are faced with an overwhelming amount of data. Lahlafi (2007) suggests that the process of searching the literature can be made easier and more fruitful if the reviewer can identify the main ideas or concepts that underpin the purpose or research question and further categorise these into keywords. She also suggests being strategic and identifying which databases or other literature sources will be beneficial to the search.

Most databases are similar in their applications, although there are some minor variations. EBSCOhost offers access to several databases. When a database such as CINAHL is accessed the searcher is presented with a screen that offers a number of choices, which are available for selection under the find box. The simplest method of searching is using a 'basic search', which involves inserting a search term (keyword or phrase) into the 'find' field and pressing 'search'. The search can be limited or expanded by pressing 'search options'. The latter presents a drop down tab that allows for phrase or individual term searching. The disadvantage of a basic search is that the database often regards phrases as individual keywords and may search for these words individually as well as in combination, which can result in a substantial number of hits of which a large number may not be relevant. An alternative option is an 'advanced search'. In this search mode the searcher is offered the option of including up to 12 other search terms that can be used to limit or expand the search. This expansion or limitation of the search is achieved through the use of Boolean operators, which are discussed later in this chapter. In the advanced search, the search terms can be refined by selecting a field within which to search that term – for example, the search term could be a name, in which case the defining field may be 'author'. This can be particularly useful if there is a known author who writes prolifically on a topic. Other search options are also available in the advanced search mode.

The next stage is to combine the searches that have been done. The searcher in this instance selects 'search history' and all the searches undertaken during this session are presented. The searcher then selects which searches are to be combined and how. This is again done using Boolean operators.

Keywords are words, terms or phrases that are used by database providers to index the works that they have stored. Through the use of appropriate keywords the database can identify what literature is being sought and so display works that are relevant. Multiple terms are used when indexing literature in a database, so the more relevant keywords that can be identified the greater the likelihood of accessing the most significant literature. Different databases use different indexing terms, which further highlights the need to identify as many relevant terms as possible. Most databases do offer a lexicon or thesaurus of indexing terms to help the reviewer identify the most applicable terms – for example, MEDLINE/PubMed use MeSH (Medical Subject Headings) when indexing articles. However, it is still worth brainstorming with subject experts, clinical colleagues and others in order to identify alternate keywords. For example, if the topic of interest was related to decubitus ulcer formation, other key words to consider would include 'pressure sores' and 'pressure ulcer' in order to identify and access some of the less recent material (Cronin et al., 2008). Another useful means of identifying keywords or phrases is to look at any articles that are available on the topic, as authors are usually asked to identify the keywords that relate to their work. Look also at keywords used by authors for their searches. Some of these may have already been identified but other alternatives may arise.

—— **Keywords unlock the database so that the relevant literature can be accessed.** ——

Another consideration with keywords is language and spelling. CINAHL and MEDLINE are both American databases, so the spelling of certain words will differ from the British English spelling. When using words such as oesophagus (esophagus), haemoglobin (hemoglobin), or tumour (tumor) it is s best to use both spellings of the word. Although most databases now employ word recognition software, which has the ability to identify potential keywords, it is always a good idea to be certain in case the alternate spelling is coded separately.

Keyword searches can be further developed through the use of commands known as Boolean operators, which are used to combine keywords so as to select or exclude articles that have the identified key words. The most frequently used Boolean operators are OR, AND and NOT and should be used as block capitals.

————————— **The most common Boolean operators are OR, AND and NOT.** —————————

The Boolean OR is used to expand a search by including more than one keyword in the same search; for example 'alcohol abuse' and 'poverty' may be combined thus:

'alcohol abuse' OR 'poverty'.

The result will identify works that contain the keywords 'alcohol abuse' or 'poverty', but not necessarily together. Alternatively AND would restrict this search to works that contained both terms, but would not include either term individually. Finally, if it was decided that the search should be restricted to adults, NOT may be used like this:

'alcohol abuse' AND 'poverty' NOT 'adolescence'.

This will identify works that contain both 'alcohol abuse' and 'poverty' but not if they contain the keyword 'adolescence' (Table 4.2).

Table 4.2   Using Boolean Operators (CINAHL search undertaken 20 December 2011)

Keywords	Hits
'alcohol abuse'	6,380
'poverty'	13,292
'alcohol abuse' OR 'poverty'	19,581
'alcohol abuse' AND 'poverty'	91
'alcohol abuse' AND 'poverty' NOT 'adolescence'	57

Another strategy that can aid in keyword searches is truncation, which involves using the root of a keyword to identify other possible forms of the word and include them in the search. Using CINAHL, by including an asterisk with the word 'diet*' the database will also search 'dietary' and 'dietetic', but can also include other terms such as 'dietician', which may not be wanted. Another search aid linked to truncation are wild cards. In CINAHL a question mark can be used to replace a letter. The database will then seek this word with every alternative letter replacing the question mark – for example, 'wom?n' will result in the search using 'woman' and 'women'. Another wild card is # which can be used for alternative spellings where a letter may or may not exist – for example, 'tumo#r' will search using both 'tumour' and 'tumor'. While the Boolean operators identified are available in most databases, truncation and wildcards do vary between databases. It is always a good idea to seek advice from a librarian who will be best placed to offer advice. Alternatively, most databases have help features that, when accessed, will guide the user through the use of these strategies.

Limiting the Search

Searches can sometimes produce a large number of hits despite the main concepts being focused. This can be particularly problematic where the word count in an assignment is restricted or there is a short time frame in which the work must be submitted. In this situation, limiting the search can reduce the number of hits to a more manageable number. While Boolean operators can be used to restrict the identified keywords or phrases, there are a number of other ways of limiting a search. One of the most commonly used limits is the age of the study. It is generally accepted that for academic assignments the studies in the review should generally be within the last five to ten years. Exceptions to this are works that are considered to be seminal or influential in the field. Alternatively, if the topic under review has been the subject of only a small number of recent studies, older works may need to be included. In this instance, however, the rationale for including the older studies should be acknowledged.

When undertaking a literature review, the vast majority of the works included should be research studies. While literature reviews, opinion articles and editorials may be helpful in identifying literature and setting the scene, the works being reviewed should be mainly research based. Limiting a search to peer reviewed research studies can be a useful way of controlling the number of identified works.

Another common means of limiting a search is in regard to language. Depending on the database used, studies published in any number of languages may be accessed, but may not be of use if there is no means of translating them. It is not unusual to see searches limited to the English language for this reason.

The above are only a few of the available methods of limiting or narrowing a search. When using these tools it is important to consider the outcome. Limiting a search to full text availability, for instance, may seem sensible if you only have access to those journals that are available on a particular database; however, colleges usually subscribe to numerous online journals, some of which may not be available as full text on the databases you are searching. By limiting your search to only full text you could lose the opportunity to review these articles. Limiting your search to studies with abstracts, however, can be very useful as you can then check how relevant these articles are before you download or search the college online journals for them.

Evaluating the Search Strategy

When doing a search for data, it is important to regularly evaluate how well the strategy being employed is working. It is unusual to be completely successful on a first search, so it is useful to review the phrases and keywords used to see how effective they were in identifying the appropriate articles. It may be that some keywords or phrases need to be further refined as they are presently too broad and getting to many results, or are identifying results that appear unrelated to the topic being reviewed. If too few useful results are being received it may be the keywords or phrases being used are too narrowly focused, or it may be that that particular database is not the most suitable one for what is being sought.

Summary

The aim of this chapter was to lead the novice reviewer through the first stages of undertaking a literature review, from identifying a problem/topic of interest through the process of doing a literature search. A number of sources from where the topic could arise were identified, one of the most popular sources being professional/clinical practice. Once the topic was identified the importance of refining the topic to make the search more manageable was discussed. The next step was to identify appropriate keywords or phrases that could be used to search for literature. The most commonly used sources of literature today are the professional databases and the Internet. Nonetheless, there are other sources and ways of searching, and these are both useful and essential in some instances. When undertaking the search it may be necessary to expand or narrow the search parameters, depending on the success of the search, and some methods of limiting the search and the use of Boolean operators were identified. Evaluating progress in the search is important as modifications to the search invariably have to be made and it is better to do this early to improve results. Remember that searching the literature is a skill and it may not always be possible to identify articles on a topic; that is not to say they do not exist, it may be simply that the wrong search term was used. It is important, therefore, to recognise that 'not being able to identify any studies' related to a particular topic is not the same as saying 'there are no studies' on that topic. The latter statement is probably wrong.

Once the literature has been found the next stage is sorting the literature to see how relevant it is and organising it so that the articles are categorised in some ordered way for easy access. This will be discussed in Chapter 5.

Key Points

- Identifying the review topic or the problem to which you are seeking a solution is the first, and probably the most important, step in undertaking a literature review.
- Literature reviews can become unfocused and unwieldy if the review topic is too broad. It is therefore necessary to refine the topic to make it more focused and manageable.
- Literature for the review should be identified and selected in a systematic manner. Databases and other sources of literature should be identified as well as the key words and search strategies that were employed.
- It is important to continuously evaluate your strategy to ensure the data that you are gathering matches the purpose of your review.

5

Reading and Organising the Literature

Introduction

This chapter considers the importance of identifying literature that is relevant to the purpose of your literature review. It outlines strategies for reading and summarising the literature effectively with a view to producing a finished piece of work that is concise and comprehensive. It offers guidance on the use of bibliographical software packages whilst discussing how the literature may be organised to aid easy retrieval once it comes to the writing-up stage.

☑ **Learning Outcomes** ☑

By the end of this chapter you should be able to:

- identify literature that is relevant to your topic.
- read and summarise the literature effectively.
- organise your literature for easy retrieval for when you come to write the review.

Identifying Literature of Interest: Selecting Appropriate Papers

A key step to identifying relevant literature is to have firstly decided on your research question. Once you have this firmly established then the task of identifying the type of literature needed becomes more focused. It is prudent to keep your question in a prominent place at all times to avoid deviating from the precise topic. The aim of undertaking a focused review of the literature is to provide information that is relevant to your topic in question.

Once you have done this, the next step is to critically evaluate pre-existing knowledge on that particular topic, whilst building upon that knowledge by identifying gaps and inconsistencies that you discover as you read. Many different types of literature will present themselves as you do your literature search. Theoretical literature typically explores relationships between different concepts that have been developed and refined over time, producing a theory that may be further challenged or tested.

Aveyard (2010) distinguishes between theoretical literature and research literature. Research literature generally involves a structured investigation that has been undertaken with the intention of answering a specific question. Research literature adopts a systematic approach to investigation and its format includes distinct sections pertaining to the aims of the study, methods used, results obtained, a discussion of the findings and recommendations. Literature in the form of discussion papers and policy documents related to practice may also be useful, depending on the purpose of your review. Practice and policy literature is usually based on up-to-date research evidence, which may be used to develop guidelines for practice (Aveyard, 2010).

A well-defined research question will guide the often difficult and time-consuming process of selecting relevant literature. If the research question is concerned with theory or policy development, then theoretical and policy literature will be the most useful source for answering the question. If the question is practice based then it is likely that research literature will be most relevant.

In order to critically appraise literature that is relevant for the review, it is important that the different types of research designs are understood. Quantitative research is primarily concerned with systematically gathering objective evidence through the use of formal instruments. The information gleaned is measured and analysed statistically. Quantitative research gathers empirical evidence that is rooted in the positivist, scientific method and adheres to a systematic and structured approach to acquiring information (Polit and Beck, 2006). Data are usually collected through the use of questionnaires, surveys and clinical trials.

In contrast, qualitative designs adopt what is known as a naturalistic approach to inquiry. This type of investigation is concerned with the understanding of subjective human experiences as perceived by the individuals participating in the research. Qualitative designs subscribe to the notion of multiple realities that are constructed by individuals and are contextually framed. Data are not measured numerically and are usually collected through interviews, focus groups and observation. Instruments for analysing the different research designs will be discussed in more detail in Chapter 6. When identifying relevant literature for your review, it is necessary to be aware of the different approaches used to answer different types of questions, and here we revert to the importance of your own research question.

Box 5.1   Reflecting on Your Research Question

If your topic of interest is, for example, the psychological phenomenon of 'hope', what type of literature will be most relevant to your review? The concept of 'hope' is in itself very broad. Is it 'hope' following a diagnosis of cancer, hope following bereavement,

(Continued)

(Continued)

or what? What is your question? If, say, you wish to explore the concept of 'hope' in women six months following mastectomy then your review is becoming more focused. It is likely that you will encounter a wide range of literature pertaining to hope but you need to remain focused on your question. As it is difficult to quantify or measure, or to attach numerical values to the concept of hope, the literature relevant to your research will more than likely focus on the complexities of human experience and perception and will be predominantly qualitative in nature.

When identifying content that is pertinent to the review, it is important to keep in mind the purpose and significance of your review. If the purpose is to serve as the basis for a research study, then the proposed investigation must be linked to the current body of knowledge on the topic and the literature review should create an argument or justification for the study (Streubert Speziale and Carpenter, 2007). Ridley (2008) suggests that it is necessary, firstly, to think about information that has to be included in the review, rather than how it is to be presented. For example, does your review have a historical context that is important for you to include? Are there any theoretical or conceptual frameworks underpinning your research question? If so, then these should be identified and included. Initially, when you start to search the literature your research question may be subject to change as you are exposed to many different types of literature.

As you progress, the relevant literature you uncover will serve to increase your understanding of the topic and you will become more astute as to what to include and what to ignore. It is your research question that provides this direction.

Reading and Summarising the Literature

As you read you will be confronted by a plethora of material, and it is essential to be able to critically appraise the content of an article in order to make a judgement as to whether or not it is worthy to include in your review. Reading with a critical eye and critiquing and analysing literature will be discussed in detail in Chapter 6. Cormack (1996) offers useful advice on how to read research reports effectively. Research articles typically follow a standard format, thereby enabling the reader to scan an article in a systematic manner and evaluate its usefulness. Being aware of the key parts of a research article – for example methods, findings, discussion and recommendations – will direct you to the sections of the report that are likely to yield important information and will alert you to its suitability for inclusion or otherwise (Benton and Cormack, 1996). Reading for academic purposes requires the student to put together information gleaned from various sources in a logical, coherent manner. It is often tempting at the outset to read everything to hand. However, this is time consuming and your reading needs to be purposeful in order to yield the information you require. As it is easy to get off track, you should be disciplined about reading only what is relevant and know how it is going to contribute to your literature review.

Avoid getting sidetracked by extraneous material that serves no purpose. Copious amounts of references do not necessarily mean a good piece of work, and it is important that your literature is relevant (Hardy and Ramjeet, 2005). As you read, you may acquire a vast amount of literature that you have difficulty in making sense of. At the preliminary stage, it is useful to skim the literature by reading the abstract, introduction and discussion sections only. This will give you an initial understanding of the key concepts that underlie each piece of work. This first impression is important as it will give you an indication of the value of the literature, while saving time that might be wasted reading irrelevant articles. As you read and reread, you will become more critical in your approach and will be able to differentiate between what is relevant and what is not. Reading at a deeper level allows connections to be made within the literature, as themes and similarities become apparent. At this point, more specific information is required and your reading needs to become more focused. Questions to ask yourself whilst reading are:

- What is the author's purpose?
- Is the problem clearly identified?
- Is there an obvious theoretical background?
- Does the author make a convincing argument?
- Are generalisations made?
- What is the significance of the study?
- Are the results presented and analysed effectively?
- Are the findings convincing?

As you read further, you are not only looking at the findings but are comparing and contrasting other findings, looking for similarities and differences and relationships within the literature. At this stage, you may be able to identify key points that relate to your own research question. This will allow you to situate your topic in the context of what you have read. When reading, it is important to devise a note-taking system. This allows for information to be organised and is useful for identifying main points. Headings may also be useful when it is proving difficult to organise and make sense of what you have read. A heading could be a subsection of your research question or topic, whereby you can group all the articles or books relevant to that section in one place, for example, using different pages for each section. Headings used in an ordered manner will ultimately help the literature review flow in a logical sequence. Using diagrams or mind maps can also allow you to see relationships between ideas or themes emerging from the literature.

Specific reading techniques have been developed to assist in reading academic literature. Shields (2010) proposes the SQ3R Reading Technique as being a useful strategy for students reading academic texts. This involves five steps: Survey, Question, Read, Recall and Review.

Survey: This involves acquiring an overview of the text by scanning it for content. Reading the abstract, introduction and conclusion gives a general idea as to the main thrust of the article. Skimming the main headings and sub-headings provides information on the main points of the text.

This initial-step survey provides a general overview of what is contained in the article and will give you an indication of its appropriateness for your own review.

Question: This step requires you to ask questions about what you have read so far. Does the article relate to your topic? Are the headings and sub-headings relevant and how do they pertain to your research question? Are any new areas emerging from the literature?

Read: Here you need to find answers to the questions you have posed. Read the article again, keeping your own topic in mind. Summarise or paraphrase the content. Taking short notes may also be useful at this stage.

Recall: In your own words, recall what you have read, referring to the questions you have posed. This helps with concentration and focuses the mind on reading.

Review: The first two Rs are concerned with understanding the content. The third R permits you to review what has been read in a more in-depth fashion. This stage facilitates an interaction with the text, allowing you to make connections with your own questions and what you have read. Making more detailed notes at this stage enables you to make comparisons with other literature and can also alert you to possible areas that warrant further investigation.

The SQ3R Reading Technique aims to promote organised and focused reading. While it may appear labour intensive at first, it is a useful strategy for learning to read effectively and purposefully. It encourages questioning and analysis and allows connections to be made between new knowledge and existing knowledge. This is a worthwhile step to undertake and can provide valuable information for the analysis and synthesis stage of the literature review.

Cohen (1990) also recommends the PQRS system (Preview, Question, Read, Summarise) as a useful tool for adding structure and focus to the reading process. Following a preview of the articles you have acquired, it is then necessary to ask questions of each paper. Cronin et al. (2008) propose CASP (Critical Appraisal Skills Programme, www.caspinternational.org) as being a useful method in the appraisal of research studies. This employs the use of different checklists that enable the user to evaluate and make sense of different types of research. An indexing or summary system can be used at the question stage (Patrick and Munroe, 2004). This involves noting the title of the article, the author, aims of the study, methodology used, findings and recommendations. The source and reference should also be included as this will enable easy retrieval of references when you come to write the review. Noting your comments about what you have read and the key points of the article is also important at this stage. This will allow you to get an overview of the literature at a glance and is particularly useful for organising and summarising your findings. It can assist in identifying similar findings or inconsistencies in the literature, which can then be elaborated on and discussed in the main body of the review.

Oermann et al. (2006) suggest IMRAD (Introduction, Methods, Results, Discussion) as being a helpful format for organising research findings. These headings can be an effective way of summarising the literature in the initial reading stage and provide a way of organising what has been read.

Devise a framework for summarising your literature. This should include your research topic and question as a starting point. Decide on the other relevant points to include, such as the source and reference of the paper and its purpose, the type of study and its relevance to your literature review, the methodology used, major findings and limitations, and your own key points and comments.

Organising the Literature

Managing a large amount of information can be a daunting task and it is important to devise a system of filing articles and references. It may be helpful to organise your literature by topic or sub-topic in order to determine how relevant each piece is to your review. If the literature is organised in a systematic manner from the outset then it will be easier to retrieve when you come to writing the review. Making notes on file cards is often a good idea as they are easier to organise and store than separate sheets of paper. As you proceed with your note taking, you will become aware of differences and similarities in the information. This will alert you to connections or relationships in the literature. Keep your notes and reference information together so that when you come to the writing stage your notes will already be organised. It is important to write out the complete bibliographic reference for each piece of work on each card.

This will make the sorting and retrieval process less problematic. Organise your notes so that all articles regarding a specific idea or theme are grouped together. This will make it easier for you when you come to critiquing the material.

Note Taking

How you take notes is a matter of personal choice. Ridley (2008) suggests three methods: annotating a hard copy of a text, pattern notes and linear notes (Ridley, 2008: 51). Annotating a hard copy of a text involves using a highlighter pen to highlight important points. Key words may be written in the margins to denote significant issues. Different colours can be used for different themes and your own comments. Pattern notes typically involve using diagrams or mind maps, where the main idea is drawn in the centre of a page, with themes and sub-themes branching out from it. Linear notes use headings and sub-headings to illustrate the important points (Ridley, 2008). Reading and note taking are interconnected. While you are reading, notes should be taken, summarising the main points. Using key words to identify important points will help you make connections between papers and references. These can then be organised into distinct categories, which will give structure to the review. If you are reviewing how a topic has developed over time, then reviewing the literature in chronological order is a good way to organise it.

Using Bibliographical Software Packages

There are many computer software packages available for use when organising your literature review (Tait and Slater, 1999; Beechcroft et al., 2006). Reference managing packages allow you to store, organise and cross-link references, insert citations and create bibliographies in different formats. Examples include EndNote (www.endnote. com), Procite (www.procite.com) and Reference Manager (www.refman.com).

Software packages such as these allow references to be downloaded from electronic catalogues and libraries and inserted directly into the text. As you write, citations can be included into the text. Your personal notes regarding your references may also be inputted into these packages. Many of these systems allow you to store your search strategy online and are valuable for retrieving search terms and references for when you come to writing the review. Specific training is usually available for these packages. It is important to mention that whatever system you use, be it manually recording references on file cards, using a software package or typing them into a word document, keeping a backup is essential. Develop the habit of keeping an up-to-date backup of your work from an early stage. References should be recorded in full as they are obtained to avoid losing information. Attention to organisation at the outset will prevent much frustration when you come to write!

Summary

Reading and organising the literature is a skill, and at times your own personal style will be challenged. However, it is important to get into the habit of doing this in an organised and structured way from the beginning. This chapter has examined how to firstly identify literature that is relevant for your review.

You will acquire a large amount of literature and it is essential to determine its relevance. The importance of determining your research question has been emphasised. This will enable you to be selective and decisive about the literature you choose to incorporate in the review. Reading and summarising the literature may often seem an overwhelming task. This chapter offers advice on how to read efficiently and effectively. Reading at a superficial level is required at first to determine the appropriateness of the literature. As you progress to a deeper level, your reading should become more critical as you start to take notes and summarise what you have read. Note taking is an important step in the reading process and is vital for organising large amounts of literature into coherent sections. Effectively managing and storing references at the outset is equally important. Methods of note taking and reference management have been outlined and discussed.

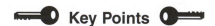 **Key Points**

- Your research question is an integral part of keeping your work focused.
- The literature you include in your review should relate to your specific question.
- Literature should be skim-read first to determine its general purpose and relevance.
- Taking notes is an important part of summarising the literature.
- Defining key terms during the summarising process will enable you to identify trends or patterns in the literature.
- Group similar studies together when organising the literature. This will allow you to see relationships between studies.
- Similarities or differences in the literature will be important for you to address as you write the review.
- It is necessary to develop a system for organising and managing your literature and references from an early stage.
- Always keep an up-to-date backup of your work.

6

Critically Analysing the Literature

Introduction

After identifying a problem or topic of interest, searching the literature and selecting the studies that appear to meet the parameters of your review, the next step is to consider how these studies will be presented to the reader. Studies within a review need to be analysed so that papers with similar outcomes can be identified, and alternative findings recognised and acknowledged. Studies are usually grouped based on these commonalities; otherwise the review risks becoming a rambling collection of isolated research studies.

The studies in the review will be presented to the reader as secondary sources, so the reader is dependent on you, the reviewer, to identify those studies that are robust, and those studies that have limitations and whose results should be read with caution. It is, therefore, essential that you can determine what strengths and weaknesses a study has in order to present them to the reader.

There is no such thing as the perfect research study. Every research study has limitations. It is expected that the strengths of a study will exceed its limitations, in which case the study is usually regarded as being good.

☑ Learning Outcomes ☑

By the end of this chapter you should be able to:

- compare and contrast findings in the literature.
- critique quantitative and qualitative research, and systematic reviews.
- analyse non-research literature.
- present critical analysis within a literature review.

Comparing and Contrasting Findings in the Literature

Having completed the literature search and organised your literature, you will probably find that you have a large number of studies that need to be presented but only
a minimal number of words in which to do this. It is important, therefore, to have
some form of structure in which to organise these studies. Having read studies related
to your topic of interest and organised your literature for retrieval, you will probably
have identified some of the themes that could be used to present your review. Themes
usually consist of studies that have related findings that can be organised into headings and sub-headings for your review. As studies often have more than one research
question or hypothesis, they may be included under more than one heading.

Once the headings have been identified, it is important to ensure that the studies
you include in that section relate to the heading. Quite often, novice reviewers can
include studies not directly related to that heading and find they have moved off on a
tangent from the original theme. It is important, therefore, to constantly compare the
findings being discussed with the heading. If the literature under a particular heading
tends to be leading in multiple directions, it may be that the heading is too broad and
needs to be refined. An alternative may be to introduce sub-headings for the smaller
themes. However, too many headings/sub-headings do mean that all the sections
will be shorter, and this can reduce the depth of analysis and discussion, which may
weaken the review. This is particularly the case where strict word limits are applied.

As mentioned earlier, headings are based around the findings and outcomes of
studies, so studies should be compared and contrasted in relation to these. It is
usual to group studies that appear to support each other together and compare and
contrast their populations and samples, methodologies and findings. Populations
are important as they can show the similarity or diversity that exists in the cohorts
included in the studies. Sample size and adherence to methodological principles
can offer an insight into the robustness of the individual studies. It is important to
remember that research should not be taken at face value and should be critically
analysed so the reader can make an informed judgement.

As well as presenting studies that support each other, it is also important to present
studies with alternative findings. Reviews should be about presenting both sides of
the debate so that the reader is informed. Studies that have alternative findings are
not necessarily inaccurate and, in fact, because they may have a larger sample size or
perhaps due to the use of a more appropriate methodology, may be more accurate
in their findings. It is, therefore, important that the reviewer can critically review
the methodologies used when comparing studies on both sides of the debate and
perhaps offer a rationale as to why the findings appear to differ.

Critiquing Research

Research studies are critiqued to identify their strengths and limitations. Just because
a study appears in a journal does not mean that its findings are accurate or that the
research has been undertaken in a robust manner. Research is one field in which all
that glitters is not always gold, so it is wiser to always read articles with a critical perspective and never accept studies at face value. There is a difference, however, between
critically reading or reviewing a study and criticising it. Seeking only limitations is

criticism and might be regarded as disapproval of the study, which is a subjective response or an admonition of the author. Alternatively, a critique is regarded as an impersonal, objective appraisal of the strengths and weaknesses of the study. It is not in any way a comment on the author's ability (Coughlan et al., 2007). This form of analysis, where the focus is on the work being reviewed, rather than the author's ability, is called an intellectual critique (Burns and Grove, 2007).

———————— **A critique is an evaluation of a study – not a criticism** ————————

A critique of a study usually looks at all the steps in the research process undertaken by the researcher when performing a study and compares these to what is generally regarded as the accepted standard. This type of critique is usually comprehensive in nature and considers such factors as the organisation and presentation of the study, the literature review, methodological issues, findings and discussion (Polit and Beck, 2012). However, when critically analysing studies in a literature review, the analysis will not be in the form of comprehensive critiques, otherwise the review would simply be a series of critiques. Rather, the analysis identifies one or two important strengths and/or limitations that will allow the reader to make a judgement on that study. Guidelines for undertaking a comprehensive critique are included here to allow the reader the opportunity to consider the full spectrum of elements that can be considered when appraising the strengths and limitations of a study.

There are a number of tools available for critiquing research studies. Some of these instruments were developed to critique both quantitative and qualitative studies, while others were developed to critique either quantitative or qualitative research. Lee (2006) and Ryan et al. (2007) query the validity of tools that attempt to critique both quantitative and qualitative research studies, claiming that the paradigms and the philosophical underpinnings that guide the methodologies are too different, and recommend separate tools for the two paradigms. Tools for evaluating different methods within the paradigms also exist. The Critical Appraisal Skills Programme (CASP), for example, offers a number of tools to assist a reviewer to evaluate different research designs such as randomised controlled trials (RCT) and cohort studies, as well as a tool for qualitative studies (CASP, 2010).

Critiquing Quantitative Research

There are numerous instruments available for critiquing quantitative research. Most research textbooks offer their own instruments, while numerous others are to be found in research journals. However, while these instruments are based on the same principles and ask similar questions, some questions are more important than others, especially in relation to evaluating a study for a literature review. When critically analysing a study in a literature review the questions that are most likely to be of importance are those that focus on the integrity or robustness of the study (Ryan-Wenger, 1992; Coughlan et al., 2007). However, for the sake of completeness, those questions that focus on the credibility of the study will also be included. When using an instrument to critique a study it is best to read through the study once or twice and become familiar with the content before beginning the critique.

Questions Related to Credibility in Quantitative Research

Credibility or believability questions (Ryan-Wenger, 1992; Coughlan et al., 2007) are usually presented first in a critiquing tool. These questions focus on aspects of the work, such as writing style, the author's qualifications, the title of the work and the abstract. These questions can be useful when critiquing a study as they can offer the reviewer some indication as to how well the study might have been conducted. A common error that is made by students or novices in the art of critiquing is to state that a study is 'weak' based on credibility variables. These questions do not look at the robustness of the study, so while these questions may lead to a first impression, judgements should be reserved until the questions related to the integrity of the study are appraised.

In considering these questions you should regard them as stimulating inquiry. So rather than simply responding with a yes or no, you should reflect on the potential implications of the researcher's action and whether this appears to strengthen or limit the credibility or the integrity of the study, depending on which factors and questions are being reviewed (see Table 6.1).

Table 6.1   Credibility and Integrity Factors in a Quantitative Research Study

Credibility/Believability: Influencing Factors and Related Questions	
Author	Do the author's experiences and/or qualifications suggest knowledge or expertise in this particular field of enquiry?
Writing style	Is the report on the study presented in a clear and organised manner? Is it easy to read and understand, grammatically correct and does it avoid excessive use of jargon?
Title	Does the report title identify what the study is about in a clear and unambiguous way?
Abstract	Is an outline of the study clearly present? Does it include the research problem, sampling method and size, methodology, findings and recommendations?
Integrity/Robustness: Influencing Factors and Related Questions	
Logical consistency	Is the study presented in a logical order following the steps of the research process?
Research problem/purpose	Is the purpose of the study or the research problem clearly defined?
Review of the literature	Is the literature review presented in an organised manner, demonstrating development of themes from previous research? Does the review offer a balanced overview of the research problem/topic of interest? Is there evidence of critical analysis of the works presented? Is the literature mainly from primary sources and is it mainly empirical or theoretical in nature?

Integrity/Robustness: Influencing Factors and Related Questions

---

Theoretical framework	Has a conceptual framework been identified? If yes, is it clearly described and is it an appropriate framework for this study?
Aims, objectives, research questions, hypotheses	Have the aims or objectives, research questions and hypotheses been presented in a clear and concise manner? Do they reflect the purpose of the study/research problem and the information gleaned from the literature review?
Research design and instruments	Has the research methodology and the rationale for selecting it been discussed? Has the research instrument been described? Is it appropriate for this study? How was it developed? Were reliability and validity testing performed? Were the results of these discussed? Was a pilot study performed?
Operational definitions	Have all the terms, theories and concepts that may influence the study been defined and clearly described to the reader?
Sample	Was the target population described? Was the method of sample selection described? Was a probability or non-probability sampling technique used? Was the sample size adequate? Were inclusion/exclusion criteria identified?
Ethical considerations	Were participants given enough information to make an informed choice in regard to participating in the study? Was confidentiality/anonymity guaranteed by the researcher? Were the participants protected from harm? Was ethical approval granted for this study?
Findings/data analysis	Were the data obtained and statistical analysis undertaken appropriate for the study? How many of the sample participated in the study? Were the data tables/charts accurate? Was the statistical significance of the findings identified?
Discussion	Were the findings discussed with reference to the literature review? If there was a hypothesis, was it supported or rejected? Did the author(s) discuss the strengths and limitations of the study? Were recommendations for future studies identified?
References	Were all the texts, journal articles, websites and other media sources referred to in the study accurately referenced?

Source: Adapted from M. Coughlan, P. Cronin and F. Ryan (2007) 'Step-by-Step guide to critiquing research. Part 1: quantitative research', *British Journal of Nursing*, 16 (11): 658–63.

Author

The expertise and qualifications of the author(s) can be good indicators of the knowledge and skills that are being brought to the study. A background and familiarity with the topic under investigation increases the likelihood that the questions will be relevant and reflect the reality of the situation. However, novice researchers with little background in an area can still do very good research, and experienced researchers can do poor research. So never assume that because the researcher is well qualified that the study will not have limitations.

Writing Style

A research report should be written in a clear and concise style. It should be easily understood and grammatically correct, avoiding the unnecessary use of jargon. It is usually expected that quantitative reports are written in the third person, which is deemed to increase objectivity.

Title

A question frequently asked is, how long should a report title be? Titles should be long enough to give the reader sufficient information as to what the study is about but short enough to avoid confusion (Parahoo, 2006). A general rule of thumb is that they should be between 10 and 15 words in length.

Abstract

Abstracts are expected to be concise but offer enough information for the reader to determine if this study is of interest. The abstract should identify the purpose of the study, and offer an overview of the research method, sample, the main findings, conclusions and recommendations. They are usually about 150–200 words in length, but there are variations between journals, and in some journals abstracts may not be clearly identified or presented.

Questions Related to Integrity in Quantitative Research

The reasoning behind these questions is to determine how robust the study appears to be, and how thoroughly the steps in the research process were adhered to. It is within this section of a critique that the strengths or limitations of a study can be determined.

Logical Consistency

A research study should be presented in a coherent manner that indicates that the researcher(s) followed the steps in the research process. The steps should be clearly defined, with logical development as the study progresses from the research problem through the literature review and onwards (Coughlan et al., 2007).

Research Problem/Purpose

The research problem or purpose of the study is usually identified early in the work and offers the reader a broad idea of what is to be investigated. It often represents a general area of interest that may need to be further refined.

Review of the Literature

In a research study the function of a literature review is to explore and refine the research problem. Any gaps in the literature, related to the research problem, should be identified. There should be evidence that an appropriate depth and breadth of reading, related to the topic, was undertaken. While the majority of studies presented should be of recent origin, it is important that influential seminal works are also included. Seminal research can help put the study into context, so it is expected that authors will include some older studies as well as contemporary literature within the review. Studies should ideally have been published within the last five years, but this will depend on the amount of literature available that is related to the research problem. The source and the nature of literature presented are two other important considerations. The literature should come from the primary source, with secondary sourced literature being used only in exceptional circumstances. Furthermore, the literature in a review should be mainly empirical in nature rather than from anecdotal or opinion articles that are not research based.

In the introduction to the literature review it is expected that the keywords used and databases sourced in the literature search will be identified. The author then usually identifies the themes that emerged from the literature as a means of signposting how the literature will be presented. The literature presented should be critically analysed and the strengths and limitations of studies included should be identified for the reader.

Theoretical Framework

A theoretical or conceptual framework is a means of organising a study. While the terms are often used interchangeably, Polit and Beck (2012) state that where the study is constructed around a theory, the framework is theoretical; and where the study is structured around a concept, the framework is regarded as conceptual. The purpose of these frameworks is to identify the concepts/theories being studied and the relationships between them. It must be stated that while not all researchers are explicit in identifying a theoretical framework, every study has a framework (Polit and Beck, 2012). Experimental and correlational studies tend to have theoretical frameworks that are better developed, with a greater likelihood of an implicit framework being found in descriptive studies. Ideally, the theoretical framework should be explicitly stated.

Aims, Objectives, Research Questions, Hypotheses

Aims, objectives, research questions and hypotheses form a link with the original research problem or purpose. They normally reflect what was found in the literature review. These factors are usually more developed than the research problem and identify the variables of interest, their possible interrelationships and the target population (Polit and Beck, 2012). The use of these factors varies with different types of quantitative studies. In descriptive studies, aims, objectives or research questions can be used to express the focus of the research; however, in some instances, the researcher will only refer to the purpose of the study. In correlational studies, where the existence of a relationship between variables is the focus of the research, research questions and/or hypotheses (a hypothesis is the research question expressed as a statement) may be presented. In experimental, quasi-experimental studies and randomised controlled trials (RCTs) hypotheses are used to identify the variables that are being explored.

Research Design and Instruments

The terms 'research method', 'research design' and 'methodology' are often used interchangeably (Parahoo, 2006). What they describe is the blueprint for the study. The research approach selected will influence, to a large degree, how the study will be performed, the method of data gathering and the type of analysis that will be performed on the data gathered.

The researcher is expected to clearly describe the research approach that has been selected and to discuss why this method was selected. The approach selected should be congruent with the purpose of the study. The next consideration is the data-gathering instrument. Again, this needs to be appropriate for what the researcher is attempting to achieve. Depending on what the researcher is investigating, there may be research instruments available that can be purchased or used with the developer's permission. However, it may also be necessary for a researcher to develop a new instrument or to adapt a pre-existing instrument.

An important feature of any research instrument is its ability to measure what it is supposed to measure (validity) and the consistency with which it measures these variables (reliability). It is, therefore, important that the researcher assesses both the validity and the reliability of the instrument that is being used. The exception can be some of the established instruments that have been shown to have strong validity and reliability with a variety of populations. In these cases the results from appropriate previous studies, in relation to validity and reliability, should be presented. However, if the researcher has any doubts, has adapted the instrument in any way or is using it on a novel population, validity and reliability testing should be undertaken.

A pilot study can be described as field-testing an instrument to determine how well it works with a sample of the population. Items that are unclear or ambiguous, which were not noticed earlier, can be identified and rectified at this stage before the main study is undertaken. Difficulties with sample selection and sample participation can also be diagnosed and corrected. The researcher should identify if a pilot study was undertaken, the numbers involved and the response rate received, and any changes that were made as a result of this field test. Participants in the pilot study or the results of the pilot study are not usually included in the findings of the main study.

Operational Definitions

It is quite common in a study to find terms or concepts whose meanings can vary considerably between one jurisdiction and another and thus alter the reader's perception of the research. It is, therefore, necessary for the researcher to ensure that all concepts and terms mentioned within the study are clearly defined so that the reader understands what exactly is being referred to.

Sampling

In quantitative research, studies should attempt to select samples that are representative of the population so as to increase the probability of generalising the findings. In order to increase the chance of a representative sample two things are required: a probability (random) sample and an adequate sample size. Probability samples can be difficult to achieve, so researchers sometimes use non-probability samples, such as convenience sampling. Non-probability samples are less likely to be representative and this should be acknowledged by the researcher if this type of sampling is used. Sample size is important because there is always a risk that a minority group within the population might dominate the sample and skew the results. The larger the sample size the less likely this is to happen and the more likely the sample will be representative, but only if the sample is selected using a probability method.

The researcher should clearly define who the population for the study were, what method of sampling was used and what the sample size was. Inclusion and exclusion criteria should also be made explicit and, if necessary, justified.

Ethical Considerations

There are four fundamental ethical principles and four moral rules, which are closely linked to these principles, which should be adhered to in all research. These are: autonomy, beneficence, non-maleficence and justice; and veracity, fidelity, confidentiality and privacy (Beauchamp and Childress, 2009). It is expected that the researcher will identify, within the study, how these principles and rules were adhered to and what processes were put in place to protect the participants. Autonomy implies that the participant has had the opportunity to make an informed decision as to whether or not to participate within the study. This decision should be made free from any coercion or promise of reward. The principle of beneficence implies that the participant and society will benefit from the outcomes of the study. Non-maleficence implies that the research will cause no harm, either physical or psychological, to the participant. While the latter two principles may appear to be the same, they are more like the opposite sides of the same coin with a different focus. Justice implies that all individuals and groups within the study are equal, and no group or individual will be privileged or disadvantaged because of their position within society. The four moral codes are closely linked to the principle of autonomy and imply the researcher will be honest, loyal and trustworthy in dealing with participants, and respect the confidentiality and privacy of subjects whether or not they participate in the study.

The researcher should also state whether ethical approval was sought and identify the approving bodies. Hospitals and institutions will generally all have ethical committees to whom research proposals must be submitted before permission to undertake the research will be granted. In the case of third-level students, permission is usually also required from the educational institution before research can be undertaken.

Findings/Data Analysis

In the findings sections, data are analysed and should be presented to the reader in a clear and concise format. The researcher usually starts by identifying how many of the sample participated in the study, which can be an important factor in determining how generalisable the results may be (Polit and Beck, 2012). It is generally accepted that a participation rate of at least 50 per cent is needed to reduce the risk of response bias.

In quantitative research, data are analysed using statistical tests. In general, descriptive research uses descriptive statistics to present findings, whereas correlational, quasi-experimental and experimental studies use both descriptive and inferential statistics. Descriptive statistics do what the name suggests and describe the numerical findings of the study. Inferential statistics are about drawing inferences or deductions from the results. The latter can be used to demonstrate if relationships exist, or if there are differences between variables, and the degree to which these relationships/differences are a result of a chance occurrence or are potentially real – this is known as the level of significance. The lowest acceptable level of significance is usually $p \leq 0.05$. This means that the probability (p) of the result happening by chance is less than or equal to 5 times out of 100.

The researcher should identify what types of statistical tests were used in the study and the results should be presented to the reader. Tables, graphs and charts should enhance the clarity of the findings but should also be congruent with them.

Discussion

After presenting the results, the researcher now needs to place these in context for the reader. If the study had a hypothesis, the researcher should state if it was supported or rejected by the findings. He should also identify if the research question was answered and whether the aims or objectives were achieved. In the discussion section the researcher presents an explanation and an interpretation of what the results might mean. This is presented with reference to the literature that was appraised in the literature review and should be consistent with the findings presented. The implications for clinical practice should also be explored. However, caution should be advised in relation to altering practice on the basis of one study, no matter how robust. It is usually within this section that the researcher will acknowledge the strengths and limitations of the study, especially in relation to the significance of the findings and their generalisability to the target population.

The study presentation usually concludes with a summary of the research undertaken, and the current state of knowledge in relation to the topic of interest. This is usually followed by recommendations for improving the current study or for future related research.

References

The author should ensure that there is an accurate bibliographical record of all the books, articles and other media sources referred to in the study. This can be a useful resource for clarifying information or for future studies in the area.

Critiquing Qualitative Research

Qualitative research is more than simply a different way of studying a phenomenon of interest. It differs from quantitative research in a number of fundamental areas such as:

- *The nature of knowledge:* it accepts that knowledge is subjective rather than objective.
- *Holism:* a phenomenon is more than the sum of its parts and cannot be reduced to a number of variables in order to study it.
- *Generalisability:* qualitative research is interested in exploring the individual's experience rather than attempting to generalise to the sample population (Ryan et al., 2007).

It is, therefore, advisable that a qualitative critiquing tool is used when analysing a qualitative study. As in the case of critiquing quantitative research, there is a wide range of critiquing tools available for critiquing qualitative research. Most textbooks will usually offer a critiquing tool specifically aimed at qualitative research and again the principles underpinning these tools are similar. As with the critiquing tool presented for quantitative research, the factors related to the integrity of a qualitative study are most likely to offer important insights to the study. Factors and questions related to the credibility and integrity of a qualitative research study are presented in Table 6.2.

Table 6.2   Credibility and Integrity Factors in a Qualitative Research Study

Credibility/Believability: Influencing Factors and Related Questions	
Author	Do the author's experience and/or qualifications suggest knowledge or expertise in this particular field of enquiry?
Writing style	Is the report on the study presented in a clear and organised manner? Is it easily read and understood and grammatically correct, and does it avoid excessive use of jargon?
Title	Does the report title identify what the study is about in a clear and unambiguous way?
Abstract	Is an outline of the study clearly present? Does it include the research problem, sampling method and size, methodology, and findings and recommendations?
Integrity/Robustness: Influencing Factors and Related Questions	
Statement of the phenomenon of interest	Is the phenomenon of interest clearly identified? Does the research question reflect the phenomenon of interest?
Purpose/ significance of the study	Is the purpose of the study or the research problem clearly defined?

(Continued)

Table 6.2   (Continued)

Integrity/Robustness: Influencing Factors and Related Questions	
Review of the literature	Has a review of the relevant literature been undertaken? Does it reflect the philosophical underpinnings related to the qualitative method selected? Were the purposes of the review achieved?
Theoretical framework	Has a conceptual framework been identified? If yes, is it clearly described and is it an appropriate framework for this study?
Method and philosophical underpinning	Was the research method identified? Why was this approach chosen? Did the researcher explain the philosophical underpinnings of the method selected?
Sample	Was the method by which the sample was selected discussed? Was the selection method suitable for the approach used? Did the sample have the appropriate experience to inform the research?
Ethical considerations	Were participants given enough information to make an informed choice in regard to participating in the study? Was confidentiality guaranteed by the researcher? Were the participants protected from harm? Was ethical approval granted for this study?
Data collection and analysis	Were the methods for gathering data and data analysis discussed? Were these methods congruent with the research approach selected? Was data saturation achieved?
Rigour	How was the trustworthiness of the study assured? Did the researcher discuss elements such as credibility, auditability, transferability and confirmability?
Findings and discussion	Were the findings presented clearly? Were the participant quotations used appropriately to support the themes? Was the report placed in context with what was already known regarding the phenomenon? Was the research question answered or the original purpose of the study addressed?
Conclusions, implications and recommendations	Will the findings of this study be of interest to the profession? Were the implications for clinical practice identified? Were recommendations made as to how future research might develop the findings of this study?
References	Were all the texts, journal articles, websites and other media sources referred to in the study accurately referenced?

Source: Adapted from F. Ryan, M. Coughlan and P. Cronin (2007) 'Step-by-step guide to critiquing research. Part 2: qualitative research', *British Journal of Nursing*, 16 (12): 738–44.

Questions Related to Credibility and Integrity in Qualitative Research

The factors influencing, and the questions related to, the credibility of a qualitative article are similar to those discussed earlier in this chapter for quantitative research. The factors and questions related to integrity, however, differ substantially, demonstrating the differences in approach between these two paradigms. Again, it is within the integrity section that the strengths and limitations of a qualitative study can be recognised. It is important to remember that the qualitative paradigm consists of a number of different research approaches each with their own, often distinct, philosophy, processes of managing and analysing data, and their own dis-crete terminology (Ryan et al., 2007). For example, within phenomenology there are a number of philosophical variations that lead to characteristic methods of manag-ing and analysing data. Husserlian phenomenologists distance themselves from the phenomenon by 'bracketing' their views, beliefs and understandings so as to prevent these influencing their description of the participants' experience. This is in contrast to Heideggerian phenomenologists who do not believe bracketing is possible, but also use this pre-existing knowledge to help them interpret the participants' experi-ences. Ethnographic researchers use a different approach to data gathering, spend-ing large amounts of time living or working in close proximity to their subjects, as well as observing or questioning them, in order to gain insights to their culture and way of life. An example of this can be seen in the movie *Avatar*, which also demon-strates one of the potential difficulties – 'going native' (Polit and Beck, 2012), when researchers completely lose their scholarly identity in favour of group membership. Grounded theory, on the other hand, uses participants' perspectives to develop and verify a hypothesis and so develop a theory grounded in the research. However, despite these differences, there are many similarities within these approaches and there are common factors that can be critically analysed (Burns and Grove, 2007).

Statement of the Phenomenon of Interest

A phenomenon is an abstract experience such as pain or anxiety. The experience of a phenomenon can be influenced by numerous different factors and so an experi-ence could be construed as quite different by two individuals or even by the same individual under different conditions. The phenomenon to be studied should be explicitly identified and this should be reflected in the research question.

Purpose/Significance of the Study

The researcher should identify why this study is important and how it will add to the body of information that already exists. The researcher should also offer a rationale for selecting a qualitative methodology to investigate this phenomenon.

Review of the Literature

The function of the literature review in qualitative research is to identify and pre-sent what is already known regarding the phenomenon of interest. This in turn will be used to support the themes that emerge from the data. In some qualitative approaches the literature review is not undertaken until after the data are gath-ered. Two such approaches are grounded theory and phenomenology. In grounded theory, data gathering and analysis should be undertaken without being preju-diced by pre-existing influences. The purpose is to generate theory from the data gathered, so for this reason the review of the literature is undertaken after data gathering is complete and with reference to the analysed data (Polit and Beck, 2012). In phenomenology, the lived experience of the participants is the central focus of the research. Again, the researcher attempts to avoid external influences until the participants' experiences have been described or interpreted, at which stage the literature is used to support the resultant themes (Burns and Grove, 2007). Ethnographic studies often use a combination of a short overview of literature at the outset of the study to contextualise the cultural issue to be investigated, and a more in-depth review later in the study to support the data analysis (Polit and Beck, 2012).

Whether the review is undertaken at the beginning of the study or after data analysis, the researcher should identify how the review was undertaken. If the literature review is done at the beginning of the study, it should be similar in nature to a quantitative review offering a comprehensive and balanced synopsis of the studies previously undertaken, conceptual or theoretical frameworks, and themes used to form a background to the study (Ryan et al., 2007).

Theoretical Framework

Theoretical frameworks can be useful in some descriptive or exploratory qualitative studies for setting boundaries or identifying why certain aspects of a phenomenon where selected for investigation. However, in other qualitative methodologies, such as grounded theory, ethnography or phenomenology, where the purpose is to develop theory, an existing theoretical framework is not used (Ryan et al., 2007).

Method and Philosophical Underpinning

The researcher should indicate why the qualitative paradigm and the particular methodological approach were chosen. The philosophical underpinnings of the approach should also be presented. The latter are important as they are the framework that identifies how the research process should proceed, for example how participants should be selected, how data should be gathered and how analysis should be undertaken. Different qualitative methodologies have different philosophies, which are often not compatible with each other, so mixing and matching (method slurring) between the different approaches is not generally recommended. Nepal (2010) and Morse (2009) argue that there are exceptions to this, for instance when the research question cannot be fully addressed unless two qualitative methods are used. However, these methods should be clearly identified from the outset of the study, and a rationale should be included as to why this mixed method approach is justified (Nepal, 2010; Morse, 2009). It is important, therefore, that there is congruence between the philosophy and the way the research is undertaken.

Sample

When selecting a sample for a qualitative study, the researcher should attempt to ensure that the participants have experience of the phenomenon under investigation. This type of sampling, known as purposive or purposeful sampling, ensures a breadth and depth of data on the phenomenon. In grounded theory, as themes emerge the researcher may select participants with experience related to those themes. This type of selection is known as theoretical sampling. Convenience samples are also used in some qualitative studies.

Samples used in qualitative research are non-probability as there is no desire to select a representative sample. Instead, the researcher seeks to generate an in-depth knowledge of the phenomenon that reflects the participants' experiences. Samples are also usually small in size. The researcher's hope is to achieve data saturation – that is, a point where the inclusion of further participants will not lead to any new data. This should be the true determinant of a qualitative sample size; however, it is rarely achievable in small research studies.

Ethical Considerations

The ethical principles and moral codes that apply in qualitative research are similar to those in quantitative studies, as is the process of ethical approval for the research. Some areas, however, need further consideration within qualitative studies. Data gathering in the qualitative paradigm often involves in-depth interviews during which participants can often inadvertently reveal information that they had not planned to discuss, or the interview may raise topics that trigger uncomfortable or forgotten experiences. As a result, participants my not feel happy or comfortable continuing with the interview. Process consent is a method of continuously negotiating with participants to determine whether they are happy to continue or wish to discontinue the interview. The principle of non-maleficence also has a role here, as the unresolved grief or other issues that may have arisen during the interview can have a negative emotional effect on the participant. In anticipation of such an event the researcher should have some form of psychological support available for participants.

Confidentiality is another ethical issue that needs consideration. The most common methods of data gathering used in qualitative research are interview and observation, and as a result participants are known to the researcher and therefore cannot be anonymous. Also, when presenting raw data to support the themes that emerge, the researcher needs to ensure the information presented will not expose the participant to being identified.

Data Collection and Analysis

There are a number of different methods of data collection available to researchers undertaking a qualitative study, the most common of which are interview (semi-structured and unstructured), focus groups and participant observation. The method of data collection, however, should be compatible with the methodology selected and the researcher should justify why that method was selected.

In qualitative research, data collection and analysis occur concurrently. Depending on the methodology adopted, there are specific steps that the researcher is expected to undertake when analysing the data. In some instances there are instruments available to aid this process; however, the instrument should be compatible with the given philosophy. To this end, there needs to be sufficient information available for the reader to determine if the final outcome of analysis is based on the data gathered in the study.

Rigour

The researcher is expected to demonstrate to the reader that steps have been taken to ensure the trustworthiness of the analytical process. The main criteria used to evaluate rigour are credibility, dependability, transferability and confirmability. Credibility attempts to establish how accurate the researcher is when representing the participants' experiences. One method of demonstrating credibility is by asking participants to review the results of the study to see if they are consistent with their experiences. Alternatively, Koch (2006) recommends that the researcher maintains a field journal – a record of interactions, reactions and content – that can be reflected upon when analysing the data and used to justify analysis. Dependability, also known as auditability, is said to exist when there is sufficient information presented for the reader to recognise and follow the decision trail. The decision trail discusses how decisions in relation to the theoretical, methodological and analytical choices were made (Koch, 2006). Transferability, also known as applicability or fittingness, is based on the degree to which the study's findings fit into other situations that are outside the context of the study. It is said to be present when readers can apply the study's results to their own experiences or when the findings are applicable to others not involved in the study. Finally, confirmability is about offering a clear demonstration of how interpretations were made and conclusions were drawn. Koch (2006) claims that confirmability can be deemed to have been achieved if the researcher can demonstrate credibility, dependability and transferability.

Findings/Discussion

There are a number of different ways in which the findings of a qualitative research study can be presented depending on the approach selected. Nonetheless, the findings should be presented clearly and supported with extracts from the data gathered. The findings should be discussed with regard to what is known about the topic, and depending on the methodological approach a further review of the literature may have been undertaken to achieve this. The findings should also be related back to the purpose of the study or research question, and the discussion should indicate if these have been satisfactorily addressed within the study.

Conclusions/Implications/Recommendations

The results of a study should add to the existing body of knowledge on that topic. It is expected that the researcher will conclude by identifying how this study is likely to do this and what implications these findings may have for clinical practice. The researcher should also state how the findings might be further developed and/or identify other related areas that arose during the study and need further investigation.

References

As in quantitative research all works referred to in the study should be accurately referenced.

Critiquing Systematic Reviews

A systematic review, unlike a conventional narrative literature review, is considered to be scientific research in its own right (Clarke, 2006). Like a review of the literature, it uses previously completed studies related to a topic of interest. However, it is in the manner in which studies are systematically selected and managed that differentiates it from a literature review. Systematic reviews are expected to be transparent and clearly describe, ideally in advance, the way in which studies will be searched, selected and evaluated. The aim is to reduce the risk of bias to the outcome through the inclusion of all studies related to the topic, both published and unpublished. Studies do not always end up being published, perhaps due to the results not being statistically significant or because of an unfavourable outcome of the study, and omitting these could influence the findings of the review. In a systematic review the reviewers are expected to methodically seek out all studies, published and unpublished, in order to present the most accurate overview of the research (Clarke, 2006). Depending on the type of data gathered, the reviewer in a systematic review may present quantitative evidence as a narrative integration if statistical tests are inappropriate, or may statistically integrate the evidence using meta-analysis techniques (Polit and Beck, 2012). Qualitative data may be integrated using meta-synthesis (Polit and Beck, 2012). Systematic reviews are discussed in more detail in Chapter 3.

Questions Related to Integrity in Systematic Reviews

Instruments for critiquing systematic reviews are now appearing more commonly in textbooks and journals. The principles that underpin these instruments are similar. Influencing factors and questions related to the robustness of a systematic review can be seen in Table 6.3.

Research Problem/Question

The research problem and/or research question should be clearly stated as to leave no ambiguity as to what is being investigated. Any operational terms or concepts used should be defined to further assist the reader in this regard. The reviewers should also identify why this review is being undertaken and why it is important to the profession.

Search Strategy and Study Screening

Systematic reviewers are expected to undertake an exhaustive, meticulous review of the literature, and how this is accomplished can offer a good insight into the robustness of the review. The reviewers should use as many alternative perspectives as possible when undertaking the search to ensure inclusivity. Also, strategies should be identified as to how the grey literature will be searched. The databases and other

Table 6.3   Integrity Factors in a Systematic Review

Integrity/Robustness: Influencing Factors and Related Questions	
Research problem and question	Is the research problem clearly identified? Do the reviewers clearly define any terminology, concepts or phenomena identified? What are the implications of this review for the profession?
Search strategy and study screening	Was the search strategy clearly identified? Were the databases and keywords identified? Were the inclusion and exclusion criteria appropriate and were they applied in a fair and consistent manner? Did the reviewers attempt to secure any missing data from the original authors or simply exclude that study? Were studies excluded for other reasons?
Quality appraisal	Was the quality of the studies selected appraised? Did the reviewers use a recognised instrument or did they develop their own? Was the instrument appropriate? Was more than one reviewer involved in the appraisal?
Combining and summarising the data	Did the reviewers clearly identify how the evidence gathered would be combined and summarised? Was the quality of the studies suitable for the analysis used? **Meta-analysis:** Were the effects of heterogeneity discussed? Did the reviewer offer a rationale for selection of a fixed or random effects model? **Meta-synthesis:** Did the reviewers discuss how the data was managed? Was there sufficient data presented to support the reviewers' findings?
Conclusions	Do the quality and quantity of the studies adequately support the conclusion drawn? Is the evidence robust?
	Were the limitations of the review discussed? Were the implications for clinical practice clearly outlined? Were recommendations for further research discussed?
References	Were all the studies and other works used in the review correctly referenced?

data sources that were accessed should be clearly identified for the reader, as should the keywords and keyword combinations that were used.

The reviewers need to rationalise clearly the inclusion and exclusion criteria for selection of studies at the beginning of the review. Reasons for exclusion can include non-conformity with the selected study design or the age of a study. However, caution needs to be taken so that exclusion criteria do not exclude a cardinal study simply because it is, for example, in a different language. Missing data should not simply be an exclusion criterion without the reviewers first attempting to locate this information. One method of doing this is to contact the original authors of the study.

Quality Appraisal

There are instruments available to assess the quality of studies for a systematic review, for example the CASP checklist for systematic reviews (CASP, 2010). However, Clarke (2006) recommends that reviewers should identify what they consider the key components of quality for their review and develop their own guidelines, and then evaluate and describe each study on that basis. Ideally, two or more reviewers should independently appraise the studies, using the agreed guidelines. The higher the degree of inter-rater agreement, the more reliable the appraisal is deemed to be (Whittaker and Williamson, 2011).

Combining and Summarising the Data

The reviewers need to indicate how the data will be combined and presented. The data may be presented using a narrative integration, meta-analysis or meta-synthesis (Polit and Beck, 2012). Narrative integration, which involves discussing the data and the studies rather than undertaking statistical analysis, is usually used when there are multiple disparities (heterogeneity) between the studies that preclude meta-analysis (Whittaker and Williamson, 2011). The rationale for using this approach should be clearly stated by the reviewers (Polit and Beck, 2012). In meta-analysis the prevailing tenet is that studies should be individually analysed and then the individual statistical results combined. Heterogeneity can be managed through using either a fixed or random effects model. Fixed effects models treat variables in the different studies as being non-random, whereas random effects models take the view that these variables are occurring by chance. Both models have their strengths and limitations (Whittaker and Williamson, 2011), so a clear rationale for selecting either should be given.

Meta-synthesis is used to analyse qualitative systematic reviews. The results are either described or, more frequently, interpreted as the reviewers integrate and seek to identify new insights into, and greater understanding of, the phenomenon. In doing so the reviewers should identify how they combined and interpreted the data. The interpretations made should also be clearly supported by the data.

In some situations systematic reviews use a mixed methodology approach using both qualitative and quantitative studies. Analysis in such situations is possible but is more complex (Whittaker and Williamson, 2011).

Conclusions

In undertaking a systematic review, the reviewers planned and organised their screening and selection criteria, so they should now discuss how robust their methods were and how closely they adhered to them. All studies have limitations and, again, it is better if the reviewers were aware of, and identified, any limitations in their review. As with any research study, systematic reviews, in adding to the body of knowledge, often identify other areas that warrant further study or review, and the authors should identify these to the reader.

References

As in all studies, all included works should be correctly referenced for the benefit of the reader.

Analysing Non-research Literature

While the majority of the literature presented in your review will be from research studies or systematic reviews, some supporting information may come from the theoretical, philosophical, practice or policy literature. This supporting information should also be critically appraised. A useful instrument for analysing practice and policy literature is the Appraisal of Guidelines for Research and Evaluation II (AGREE II) (Brouwers et al., 2010), available at www.agreetrust.org.

Another helpful tool for critically analysing non-research literature is presented by Hek and Langton (2000). This instrument focuses on the perceived accuracy, trustworthiness and quality of the paper being reviewed. The use of this tool does require a reasonable knowledge of the subject area. Hek and Langton (2000: 51) acknowledge that the appraisal in their review was performed by 'subject knowledgeable' reviewers. An adaptation of Hek and Langton's (2000) instrument is displayed in Table 6.4.

Table 6.4   Analysing Non-research Literature

Influencing Factors and Related Questions	
Purpose and relevance	What is the aim of this article? Is it congruent with the purpose of the review?
Credibility	Is the report on the study presented in a clear and organised manner? Is it easy to read and understand and grammatically correct, and does it avoid excessive use of jargon? Does it appear credible at first glance?
Peer review	Is the article published in a peer-reviewed journal?
Supporting evidence	Do the author's experiences and/or qualifications suggest knowledge or expertise in this particular field of enquiry? Does the journal have a high impact factor?
Accuracy and reliability	Is the information presented in the article accurate? Is it congruous with the literature and what is known about the phenomenon? Is there a fit between what the author suggests and experience/knowledge of the phenomenon?

Source: Adapted from G. Hek and H. Langton (2000) 'Systematically searching and reviewing literature', *Nurse Researcher*, 7 (3): 40–57.

Presenting Critical Analysis Within a Literature Review

As stated earlier, a literature review is not a series of critiques. The focus should be on the findings of the studies and the robustness of these outcomes. The reviewer has to be able to present the reader with both the findings and the critical analysis of the study in a succinct but also an objective manner. It is, therefore, not possible to mention more than one or possibly two of the factors that influence the robustness of a study when critically analysing it. It is also important to remember at this point that critical analysis, like critiquing, is not about criticism – that is, it is not simply focused on limitations but should also highlight the strengths that studies possess. When critically analysing an influencing factor in the methodology of a study, the reviewer should also consider the implications of this strength or limitation, more specifically how it could possibly have influenced the outcome of the study.

Critical analysis, like the review itself, should always be presented in an objective manner so no personal views should be expressed. It is, therefore, imperative that the critical analysis and the implications are presented with reference to research textbooks or journal articles. This allows you, as the reviewer, to remain independent as you are only identifying the approach used by the researcher, whereas the textbook is commenting on the robustness and possible implications of the approach used.

Summary

The purpose of this chapter was to introduce the novice reviewer to the concept of analysing the literature. A literature review can consist of a large number of studies, and these need to be organised for the benefit of the reader. Studies with findings reflecting similar themes are thus identified and grouped together under headings so that the reader can consider the different perspectives and implications.

For the reader to make an informed judgement on the implications of a study, it needs to be presented in such a way that they can recognise how robust the findings of that study are. No study is perfect and not all studies are necessarily robust, even if they are in print, so the reviewer must analyse each study with a critical eye so that the reader can make an informed judgement as to the study's strengths and/or limitations.

In critically analysing a study the reviewer needs to remain impartial and use research texts or articles to support the analysis. It is also important to remember that strengths are as important as limitations, and only seeking the latter could be regarded as criticising someone's work rather than evaluating it.

The next step after analysis is synthesis – that is, the combining of data from a number of studies to create new insights or perspectives. Synthesising the literature is the focus of the next chapter.

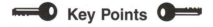 **Key Points**

- If literature is worth reviewing, it is worth reviewing critically.
- A critique or critical analysis is about identifying the strengths and/or limitations of a study; it is not about criticising the authors or their work.
- Critical analysis is undertaken in an objective manner and supported by appropriate texts and literature.
- There are a variety of different instruments available to help you critically analyse the different types of studies and literature.

7

Synthesising the Literature

Introduction

Whatever type of literature review you are undertaking, at this point in the process you will have identified and collected your literature, undertaken a quality assessment (analysis) of that literature and perhaps extracted appropriate data. The next step is to combine or pool the results, and this chapter explores the various means by which this might be done. As with many other parts of undertaking a literature review, how you will go about this is dictated by the type of review you are undertaking and the type of data (literature sources) you have included. The chapter focuses firstly on what is described as thematic analysis. This is because most undergraduates undertaking literature reviews as a stand-alone academic assignment or as a thesis chapter undertake narrative reviews with which thematic analysis is most commonly associated. However, the chapter outlines other synthesis methods often used in systematic reviews so that you have an awareness and understanding of them and where and in what situations they are used.

☑ **Learning Outcomes** ☑

By the end of this chapter you should be able to:

- explain how to summarise and present the findings of your analysis of the literature.
- describe the steps involved in synthesising the findings of your analysis of the literature.
- explain the main types of synthesis that can be undertaken.
- describe how an appropriate method of synthesis is chosen.

Presenting and Summarising Results

Regardless of the type of literature review that is being conducted, the first step of the synthesis is to present your findings. This should include a detailed presentation of your search strategy, the results of your search, the process by which literature was included or excluded and a collation of information about each study.

All contemporary literature reviews require a detailed presentation of the search strategy you conducted. These can be presented in text or tabular form, although the latter aids clarity and readability. Aspects that might be included are: the databases searched, time and language delimiters, search terms with Boolean operators, the date the search was conducted, the number of hits, the number judged to be irrelevant and discarded following review of the title, and the number retained for full review (see Table 7.1).

Most contemporary literature reviews do not confine themselves to searching online databases, and other sources such as manual searches, textbooks, catalogues, grey literature and dictionaries (see Chapter 4 for descriptions of each type of literature) are valuable sources. The results of these searches should be presented also.

In systematic reviews it is a requirement that a collation of information about each study included in the review is presented. This is referred to by Arai et al. (2009: 377) as 'descriptive synthesis'. Increasingly, this standard is being applied to narrative reviews in order to counter criticisms about their being less systematic and explicit than other approaches (Mays et al., 2005). Moreover, describing and analysing key aspects of each literature source enhances the level of synthesis and moves the review beyond a summary. Although many of the review publications in journals present a tabular summary of the research studies included in their review, it is important in a narrative review that tables are constructed for other types of literature, such as secondary sources – for example, literature/systematic reviews – and non-research literature – for example, theoretical, experiential, philosophical and

Table 7.1 Example of Tabulation of Online Database Search

	Database and Time Limits	Language	Search Date	Search Terms	Number of Hits	Number Discarded (unrelated title)	Number Reviewed (title and abstract)	Number Reviewed (full text)
Online Databases	PubMed (Unlimited)	English	01.09.12	'pancreatitis' 'pain' 'assessment' 'management' 'analgesia'	425	344	81	24
	CINAHL (1990-present)	English	10.09.12	'pancreatitis' 'pain' 'assessment' 'management' 'analgesia'	209	160	49	19

policy. This is because narrative reviews are often concerned with the current state of knowledge on a topic, and literature other than primary studies can be important for contextualising or situating the problem or focus of the review.

As part of the process of critically analysing the literature, as described in the previous chapter, you will have asked questions of each publication and extracted key information from each source. You will probably have developed or used a published template to undertake the appraisal and document the detail of each publication, and it is these individual summaries that form the basis of your overall summary. Whatever critical appraisal tool you have used, you should be able to extract the source and full reference, the title of the article, the author, the purpose and methodology used in a research study, and the findings and outcomes. It is also useful to incorporate comments or key thoughts on your response to the article after it has been reviewed.

How you decide on what should be included in your summary table is largely dependent on the type of literature you are presenting – that is, research or non-research. Other factors that you will need to consider are whether or not you are following a strict protocol, as in a systematic review, or if you are preparing a review for publication where reporting guidelines such as the Preferred Reporting Items for Systematic Reviews and Meta-analyses (PRISMA) are being used (Moher et al., 2009).

In Chapter 3 on systematic reviews, two templates based on PICO and PEO for recording information were presented. However, your literature may not easily fit within these types of templates. Alternative examples of tabular summaries for primary (research) studies are outlined in Tables 7.2 and 7.3. The first, taken from

Table 7.2   Summary Table – Example 1

Reference	Research Design	Sample	Methods	Findings
Fored et al. (2001)	Nationwide, population-based, case-control study	926 Swedish patients with newly diagnosed renal failure and 998 control subjects	Face-to-face interviews and statistical logical regression models	Aspirin and non-steroidal anti-inflammatory drugs (NSAIDS) were used regularly by 37% and 25% respectively of the patients with renal failure and by 19% and 12% respectively of the controls, supporting the exacerbating effects of NSAIDs and aspirin on chronic renal failure. However, there is possible bias because of analgesic consumption incurred by co-morbidities.
Singer et al. (1999)	Qualitative study	126 Canadian patients, comprising 48 dialysis patients, 40 patients with HIV and 38 residents of a long-term care facility	Content analysis of in-depth interviews	Participants identified pain and symptom relief, avoiding a prolonged death, having control, relieving burden and strengthening relationships with loved ones as critical for quality, end-of-life care.

Source: A. Williams and E. Manias (2008) 'A structured literature review of pain assessment and management of patients with kidney disease', *Journal of Clinical Nursing*, 17: 74–5.

Williams and Manias (2008), is a structured literature review of pain assessment and management of patients with chronic kidney disease. Whilst they included non-research literature in the review, the tabular summary presented in the publication was limited to the 12 primary studies sourced.

The literature review outlined in Table 7.3 was a narrative review of the impact of caring for those with chronic obstructive pulmonary disease (COPD) on carers' psychological well-being and consisted of 20 studies (13 quantitative, seven qualitative).

As can be seen from these examples, there are variations in the focus and detail provided. Whilst this may be due, in part, to publishing restrictions, it is evident that collating data in this way enhances the rigour of the review primarily because it enables the reader to discern the relationship between the reviewer's interpretation and the literature upon which it was based. It is recommended, however, that when you are preparing such a table for an academic assignment, as opposed to a journal publication, additional details, such as the full reference and source as well as evaluative comments, are useful.

When preparing a summary table for secondary sources such as reviews, your template will have different headings from those used for primary research. However,

Table 7.3   Summary Table – Example 2

Reference and Country of Study	Research Design and Methods	Study Aims and Objectives	Definition of Carer provided	Participants and Setting	Main Findings Relevant to the Review
Pinto et al. (2007) Brazil	Cross-sectional descriptive study Assessment tools: medical outcome survey – short form (SF-36) Caregiver Burden Scale	To determine the effect of COPD on the quality of life of carers	Yes – a person who provides most of the care required by the patient during the course of the disease and is most intimately aware of the patient's needs	42 patients who had COPD and their caregivers visiting a pulmonary outpatient department	Regression analysis showed caregiver/ patient relationship quality, SF-36 caregiver mental component summary and SF-36 patient physical component summary are important predictors of caregiver burden
Seamark et al. (2004) UK	Semi-structured interviews analysed using interpretative phenomenological analysis	To explore the experiences of patients with severe COPD	Not provided	Sample of nine men and one woman with COPD and their carers	Loss of personal liberty and dignity Distress at seeing breathlessness Adaptive strategies to cope with the disease Appreciation of continuity of care and reassurance received from healthcare professionals

Source: M. Grant, A. Cavanagh, and J. Yorke, (2012) 'The impact of caring for those with chronic obstructive pulmonary disease (COPD) on carers' psychological well-being: a narrative review', *International Journal of Nursing Studies*. DOI: 10.1016/j.ijnurstu.2012.02.010.

Table 7.4   Example 1 of Summary Table for Systematic Reviews

Reference	Research Question/ Purpose	Search Strategy, Inclusion/ Exclusion Criteria	Study Selection	Quality Assessment	Data Synthesis

as you know from the Chapter 2 on types of literature, their purpose and focus can vary considerably. Therefore, as the evaluative criteria you use will differ depending on the 'type' of review you are including so too will the headings you use to present your summary table. For example, the criteria by which you evaluate a systematic review may differ from a narrative review that is simply presenting the current state of knowledge or offering a perspective on a topic (Cronin et al., 2008). Drawing on the evaluation tool presented in Chapter 6, Table 7.4 offers an example of the headings that could be used in a summary table of systematic reviews.

An example of an alternative, based on the AMSTAR (assessment of multiple systematic reviews) instrument (Shea et al., 2007) is presented in Table 7.5. The objective of this review of systematic reviews was to identify effective training strategies for teaching communication skills to qualified physicians. Twelve systematic reviews on communication skills training programmes were included.

Deciding how to present non-research literature can be complex because it can vary considerably. Initially, as with all literature sources, it is important that you undertake a critical appraisal and that you do not just accept such literature at face value. For example, if you were undertaking a literature review about social support in persons with chronic obstructive pulmonary disease (COPD), you will have come across or sourced literature related to theories of social support. In your reading you may determine that these theories offer different perspectives or explanations of the impact of social support. Whilst a detailed analysis of each theory may be beyond the scope of your review, it is important that you explore the development of the theory and the evidence that exists to support it.

Similarly, with other non-research literature, such as policies and/or practice guidelines, you should not assume they are valid and should appraise the evidence on which they are based. While most of the published or generic critical appraisal tools that are available focus on appraising research or secondary sources, they can be adapted for use with non-research literature. Alternatively, criteria for analysing non-research literature, such as those outlined by Hek and Langton (2000) (see Chapter 6), can be used and can then form the basis of the tabular summary of your non-research literature as outlined in Table 7.6.

Depending on the nature of your review, you may choose to present additional information in tabular or diagrammatic representations that aid understanding or enhance the clarity of the review. For example, you may want to extract details such as sample sizes, types of interventions or any scoring measures that were used, such as pain scales and quality of life measures (Table 7.7).

Once you have completed the presentation and summary of your results how you progress to the next stage depends on the type of data that you have. For example, your review may contain a mixture of literature, as outlined above, or it may be confined to research studies. If it is the latter these, in turn, can be of a similar design (for example, RCTs) or a mixture of designs (qualitative and quantitative

Table 7.5   Example 2 of Summary Table for Systematic Reviews

Review	Type of Review	No. of studies	Quality of Studies Included	Type of Studies Included	Target Population	Patient Groups	Control Groups	Type of Outcome	Theoretical Background	Conclusions
Lane and Rollnick (2007)	Review	25	Not reported	RCTs	HCPs (Health Care Practitioners)	Sim patient	No training	Behavioural observation	Interactive training strategies	Outcomes were better in programmes that included skills practice than in purely didactic programmes. No significant differences were found between simulated patients and role play.
Fellowes et al. (2004)	Review	3	All studies met the criteria	RCTs	Specialists (oncology)	Real patients	No training	Objectives assessments of patients' and nurses' behaviour with validated coding strategies	Lipkin model	Two programmes were effective; one was unclear.

Source: M. Berkhof, H.J. van Rijssen, A.J.M. Schellart, J.R. Anema and A.J. van der Beek (2011) 'Effective training strategies for teaching communication skills to physicians: an overview of systematic reviews', Patient Education and Counseling, 84: 156—8.

Table 7.6   Example of Summary Table for Non-research Literature

Title	Author Year	Journal (ref)	Purpose	Credibility	Quality	Content	Coherence	Recommendations	Key Thoughts/ Comments

Table 7.7   Example of Additional Information that May Be Presented

Reference	Number of Participants	Male	Female	Age Range
Taylor (1999)	52	30	22	18–64
Brown (2004)	112	45	67	25–70
Johnson (2010)	86	52	34	22–60

data). Therefore, the most fundamental factor in what you do with your data is heterogeneity (difference), either at the level of the type of literature you have or at the level of the types of studies that are included.

Methods of Synthesis

A large number of methods of synthesis have emerged, some of which were referred to in Chapter 3. Many of these methods have emerged to manage the synthesis of particular types of data and can be crudely divided into those that address qualitative studies, quantitative studies, mixed research or mixed literature. The most prominent of these are outlined in Table 7.8, although this is not a finite or all-encompassing list. Whilst some of these are addressed later in the chapter, in order to enable you to become familiar with them, the main focus is on what is known as thematic analysis since this is the approach you are most likely to use.

Thematic Analysis

As indicated earlier, thematic analysis is the most common method for summarising and synthesising findings in a narrative review, although it is considered more basic and less rigorous than other synthesis strategies. While there is always, of necessity, a level of interpretation, the focus of thematic analysis is often on providing a summary

Table 7.8   Methods for Synthesising Data

Synthesising mixed literature	⟶ thematic analysis, narrative synthesis
Synthesising quantitative studies	⟶ meta-analysis, narrative synthesis
Synthesising qualitative studies (meta-synthesis)	⟶ meta-ethnography, meta-study, meta-narrative, qualitative meta-summary, thematic synthesis, critical interpretive synthesis and grounded theory

rather than new insights or knowledge associated with synthesis. Findings are generally preserved in their original form – that is, there is no data transformation.

The reviewer identifies and brings together the main, recurring or most important themes in a body of literature (Mays et al., 2005). However, in many of the literature reviews presented in academic assignments or in published narrative reviews, one of the things that is rarely clear is how the reviewer arrived at the said themes. To some extent, this impacts on the overall rigour of the review. Outlined below is a process that is not unlike data analysis in qualitative research, which enhances and strengthens the integrity of your review.

As indicated above and as its name suggests, the overall aim of a thematic analysis is to identify themes from the literature. In order to achieve this, it is necessary to undertake analysis in such a way that it is evident that the final themes have emerged clearly from the data (literature). In order to ensure this, the first step should be to engage in coding. Essentially, a code is a symbol or abbreviation used to classify words or phrases in the data. Simply put, a code labels and identifies the point being made in a particular piece of data. What constitutes data, and therefore what will be coded, will differ depending on the type of literature you have. For example, if you are coding a research study then your focus should be on the findings section. If you are coding non-research literature then the discussion section of the paper should be your focus. Although this may seem laborious, the findings or discussion section of each piece of literature should be examined and coded. The initial codes may alter as the process progresses and as the reviewer becomes more familiar with and more proficient at identifying appropriate codes.

Once all the relevant sections have been coded, the next step is to develop themes, which involves grouping the codes. It is advisable to begin this process by grouping codes that are the same or very similar as they are likely to be the easiest to manage. Grouping of codes that are not evidently similar presents more of a challenge and therefore takes longer. What is important here is that you keep the original articles to hand to ensure that you are remaining faithful to the findings.

You then need to label or give a name to the theme(s). The theme name should be a reflection of the codes contained therein. However, naming the theme at this stage does not preclude altering the name at a later stage. This process should proceed until all codes are assigned to a theme. Table 7.9 provides an example of a process of analysis that included 49 qualitative reports and six concept analyses in

Table 7.9   Example of Analysis in a Meta-synthesis

Codes	Sub-categories	Categories
Skills Decision-making Interpersonal skills Competence Knowledge base Experience	Nursing knowledge and skills (competence)	Professional maturity
Ability to cope Self-confidence	Professional maturity	

Source: D.L. Finfgeld-Connet, (2008) 'Meta-synthesis of caring in nursing', *Journal of Clinical Nursing*, 17: 196–204.

a meta-synthesis of caring in nursing (Finfgeld-Connett, 2008). Although different terms were used – that is, sub-categories and categories – the principles of thematic analysis remain the same.

At the end of the process, you will have findings (codes and themes) that support each other but it is important to note that you are likely also to have some that are contradictory. These similarities or differences require further scrutiny, and it is at this point that you return to your critical analyses to try to account for them. For example, the studies in your review are likely to have been conducted in different contexts or cultures, used varying research designs and/or had different sample sizes or composition. Examining these factors enables you to draw inferences about why results are different. It also offers you the basis for presenting an analytical rather than simply a descriptive account of the literature in your review because you will be able to discuss the strength of the evidence that supports any particular argument. There may also be contradictions between the findings of research studies and, for example, experts in the field. Whilst this is not unusual, you will be required to evaluate the evidence and draw conclusions as to the strength of each.

Aveyard (2010) suggests that in some situations you may not be able to account for differences in the results of studies or there may not be any real consensus. To a large degree, this 'finding' is as significant as if the literature achieved a consensus because it may point to a need for further study in the area. However, it may also mean that you are not able to provide an answer to your original review question. Documenting this process as you are undertaking it is a good idea and also helps you prepare for the writing of your review. The themes you have developed constitute your findings and will structure your subsequent discussion (see Chapter 8).

Narrative Synthesis

A short discussion of narrative synthesis is included here because of the potential for confusing it with the thematic analysis used in a narrative or traditional literature review. As indicated above, thematic analysis has been the most common method for summarising or synthesising findings in a traditional or narrative review. A narrative synthesis is similar in that it uses a narrative as opposed to a statistical approach to synthesise evidence. However, it differs essentially in its level of synthesis in that it attempts to generate new knowledge or insights (Mays et al., 2005). The narrative encompasses the analysis of the relationships within and between studies as well as providing an assessment of the strength of the evidence (CRD, 2009).

Popay et al. (2006) suggest that narrative synthesis can be used in three ways: before undertaking a statistical analysis (meta-analysis); instead of undertaking a statistical analysis where the experimental or quasi-experimental studies are too diverse to allow for meta-analysis; and where the review questions include a wide range of different research designs and research/non-research literature. To date, however, its use has been associated primarily with the synthesis of multiple studies in systematic reviews.

As part of a project for the Economic and Social Research Council (ESRC) Methods Programme, Popay et al. (2006) developed a framework for narrative synthesis that focuses largely on the effects of interventions and the factors that influence how these are implemented. Nonetheless, there appears to be potential for the framework to be applied to a range of literature. Not only do the authors argue for the flexibility and iterative (non-linear) nature of the process but within the four elements that comprise the framework (Box 7.1) 19 tools and techniques that can be used for undertaking a narrative synthesis have been proposed. The reviewer(s) choose whichever tools or techniques are most appropriate for the data that is being handled. For example, when exploring relationships within and across studies techniques such as conceptual mapping and qualitative case descriptions could be usefully applied to the results of qualitative studies while moderator variables and subgroup analysis might be employed for the findings of quantitative studies (Popay et al., 2006). Essentially, what this framework does is provide a systematic and potentially trustworthy and robust means of organising, describing and interpreting study findings for the purpose of explanation. While some of the tools and techniques are complex and beyond what would be expected for an academic assignment or literature review as part of a dissertation, there is potential to adapt or use some of them to enhance the transparency and credibility of the your review process. The authors of the framework have published two examples of how its elements can be applied (Arai et al., 2009; Rodgers et al., 2009).

Box 7.1   The Four Main Elements of Narrative Synthesis (Adapted from Popay et al., 2006)

- Developing a theory of how the intervention works, why and for whom
- Developing a preliminary synthesis:

  o Tabulations.
  o Groupings and clusters.
  o Textual descriptions.
  o Translating data.
  o Transforming data: constructing a common rubric.
  o Vote counting as a descriptive tool.

- Exploring relationships within and across studies:

  o Conceptual triangulation.
  o Reciprocal/refutational translation.
  o Investigator and methodological triangulation.
  o Moderator variables and subgroup analyses.
  o Idea webbing/conceptual mapping.
  o Qualitative case descriptions.
  o Visual representation of relationship between study characteristics and results.

- Assessing if the synthesis is robust:

  o Use of validity assessment.
  o Best evidence synthesis.
  o Checking the synthesis with authors of primary studies.
  o Reflecting critically on the synthesis process.

Meta-analysis

As outlined in Chapter 3, meta-analysis is a process of statistical analysis of numerical data the purpose of which is to pool the results of individual studies and re-analyse them as one, bigger data set. In order to undertake a meta-analysis the research designs and methods of the included studies must be reasonably homogeneous (similar) with the gold standard being RCTs. The outcome of such an exercise is to increase the power and the accuracy of the effect of an intervention, something which may not be evident from single studies. In addition, meta-analyses can also resolve controversy where there have been conflicting results or claims arising from them (Higgins and Green, 2008; CRD, 2009). However, caution must also be exercised as meta-analyses have the potential to be misleading. This may be where studies have biases or errors that render them of poor quality, and in the act of combining them they are given a level of credibility they should not have. Therefore, the review team must carefully consider biases within studies, variations across studies and any reporting biases during the review process (Higgins and Green, 2008).

Most meta-analyses are undertaken in two stages, the first being an analysis of the outcome and a calculation of summary statistics for each individual result. In the second stage, the results are pooled to give an overall summary effect (CRD, 2009). The calculated result is referred to as a 'single summary statistic' or 'effect measure' (Booth et al., 2010: 294). Simply stated, the effect measure is the observed relationship between an intervention and an outcome. Standard effect measures include: 'odds ratio', 'relative risk', 'risk difference', 'numbers needed to treat', 'standardised mean difference' and 'weighted mean difference' (Booth et al., 2010: 294). Odds ratio and relative risk are the most commonly used measures but they can only be used with dichotomous (binary) outcome data. Data are referred to as dichotomous or binary data when for every subject or participant there can only be one of two outcomes – for example, sick/well, pregnant/not pregnant. Brief definitions of odds ratio and relative risk are given in Box 7.2.

Box 7.2   Definitions of Effect Measures – Binary Data

Odds Ratio

The odds ratio is a relative measure of risk that assesses the likelihood that exposure to a factor under study will result in someone developing an outcome compared to someone who is not exposed. An odds ratio of 1 indicates no difference between the groups being compared.

Relative Risk

Relative risk compares different risk levels. Therefore, in a study where there is an intervention and a control group, the relative risk is the proportion of participants who experience an event in both groups. A relative risk of 1 indicates no difference between the groups being compared.

(Higgins and Green, 2008; Booth et al., 2010)

Effect measures for continuous data include the 'mean difference' (weighted mean difference) and the 'standardised mean difference' (Box 7.3). Continuous data is that which can have an infinite number of possible values. Weight, area and volume are true examples of continuous data but in meta-analysis the above effect measures are also applied to data such as that found in measurement scales (Higgins and Green, 2008).

Box 7.3   Definition of Effect Measures – Continuous Data

Mean Difference (Weighted Mean Difference)

The mean difference is a summary statistic that measures the absolute difference between the mean value in two groups. It estimates the amount by which the intervention changes the outcome on average when compared with the control group.

Standardised Mean Difference

The standardised mean difference is a summary statistic that signifies the extent of the effect of the intervention relative to the variability (Standard Deviation) observed in an individual study. It is used when studies have measured the same outcome but have not done so in the same way; for example, the same measurement scale has not been used. This statistic enables the results of individual studies to be standardised to a uniform scale before being combined.

As stated above, in the second stage of a meta-analysis the statistics from each individual study are 'pooled' to give an overall summary estimate (CRD, 2009). This is generally done by weighting each study estimate using what are known either as 'fixed-effect' or 'random-effect' models (Whiting, 2009). The reason for weighting the contribution of each study is that not all studies are the same in terms of how precise they are and how much information they present. It is, therefore, not possible to simply take the effect size in each study and calculate the overall mean. What the fixed-effect or random-effect models offer is a way of determining how studies are weighted. However, because these models operate under different assumptions, the manner in which studies are weighted differs. For example, the fixed-effect model, as its name suggests, assumes one effect size and it only assigns weight by virtue of the amount of information contained within each study. Thus, studies that are larger and contain more information are given more weight than smaller studies. Conversely, and as its name suggests, the random-effect model does not assume one effect size but argues that the effect can vary across studies. This can be due to factors such as the population in the study, the manner in which the intervention was implemented or even the reliability of the methodology for measuring the effect. Therefore, in a random-effect model the weighting of studies is more balanced between larger and smaller studies.

Results from a meta-analysis are commonly presented using what is known as a forest plot (Figure 7.1). A forest plot presents the results of each study within a

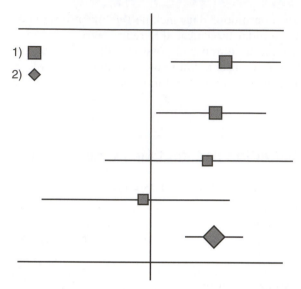

Figure 7.1   Example of a Forest Plot

review as well as the combined result of the meta-analysis. An important part of a forest plot is that it can display what is known as the confidence interval. The confidence interval, represented by a horizontal line, informs the reader about the level of uncertainty associated with each result. A wide confidence interval indicates that different results are likely to occur were the study to be repeated. The vertical line represents 'no effect', which means that there is no difference or benefit to the intervention group when compared to the control group. The overall meta-analysis result is often represented as a diamond-shape.

This brief introduction to strategies used in meta-analysis highlights the complexity of the endeavour, and any attempt at such an undertaking will, almost certainly, require the assistance of a statistician. There are also software packages that are available to help with process, notably Review Manager (RevMan) that is used for preparing and maintaining Cochrane Reviews.

Meta-synthesis

Chapter 3 on systematic reviews introduced the conception of meta-synthesis as a term that encompasses the various methods that have been developed to address the synthesis of qualitative research. As with meta-analysis, developments in meta-synthesis can be associated with the recognition that single studies may offer little in terms of having an impact on clinical practice and/or healthcare policy or research. In an era where healthcare strategy is focused on developing person-centred services, combining the results of findings from qualitative-research studies serves to enable knowledge accumulation of the needs and experiences of the patient or service-user (Ring et al., 2011).

While the focus here is on the techniques for synthesising qualitative research findings, it must be noted that proponents of the various methods of meta-synthesis have developed phases or stages for the conduct of the whole review. Yet, the same terms are used also to identify the synthesis stage of the review. The interchangeable use of terminology to define the whole process and/or the synthesis stage can be confusing for those who are new to meta-synthesis. Ring et al. (2011) identify that synthesising qualitative research is complex, due in part to the lack of consensus and continued debate about terminology and methods. What is important, however, is that the analysis and synthesis of the findings of the review are explicitly described and presented.

Methods of meta-synthesis are concerned for the most part with interpretation rather than the aggregation (adding together) that is the focus of meta-analysis. Although the process by which this is done varies, most involve deconstruction (or breaking down) of the research findings from individual studies, examination of the findings to discern the key features, following which they are combined in a transformed whole or new interpretation (Flemming, 2007; Finfgeld-Connett, 2010). Whilst numerous methods for synthesising qualitative research findings have emerged, this section will introduce meta-ethnography, meta-study and qualitative meta-summary as three distinct approaches. Meta-ethnography (Noblit and Hare, 1988) is included because it is the most commonly cited and possibly leading method for synthesising qualitative healthcare research. Meta-study (Paterson et al., 2001) is a multi-faceted approach that has three analytic phases that differentiates it from other methods. Both of these methods are oriented towards data synthesis and interpretation (Finfgeld-Connett, 2010). Qualitative meta-summary is an approach that looks to aggregate qualitative findings for the purpose of determining the frequency of each finding (Sandelowski and Barroso, 2007). Strictly speaking, because of its emphasis on aggregation and not interpretation it could be argued that it is not a form of meta-synthesis. Nonetheless, it is included here because it is a novel approach that was developed originally to address qualitative findings.

Meta-ethnography

Meta-ethnography was first proposed by Noblit and Hare (1988) in the field of education as an alternative to meta-analysis and has emerged as the leading method for synthesis of qualitative research (Ring et al., 2011). Noblit and Hare (1988) focused originally on studies that they described as ethnographic although its contemporary use has been extended to include a range of qualitative studies. The main purpose of a meta-ethnography is to create what is described as a new or third-order interpretation. First-order concepts are those identified by the participants in the original studies while second-order concepts are the interpretations made by the authors of these studies. Therefore, meta-ethnography is a synthesis of first- and second-order concepts to construct a new interpretation or theory about the phenomenon under study (Atkins et al., 2008). Whilst Noblit and Hare developed a whole method (Box 7.4) the emphasis here is on stages 4, 5 and 6 that are concerned with managing the data after it has been identified and extracted from the included studies.

Box 7.4   Meta-ethnography Method (Adapted from Noblit and Hare, 1988)

1 Getting started (determining the research question).
2 Deciding what is relevant to the initial interest (defining the focus, determining inclusion/exclusion criteria, identifying relevant studies, undertaking quality assessment).
3 Reading the studies.
4 Determining how the studies are related (creating a list of themes, concepts or metaphors, putting them side by side or close together (juxtaposing) and determining how they are related).
5 Translating studies into one another (comparing the concepts/metaphors).
6 Synthesising translations (trying to create a new, higher-order interpretation).
7 Expressing the synthesis (presenting the synthesis).

Before the studies are translated into one another in stage 5, it must first be determined how they are related. Therefore, in stage 4 of the meta-ethnography, the reviewers or meta-synthesists examine each study and construct a list of themes, concepts or metaphors that form the data for the synthesis. This is the process of deconstructing and decontextualising the study findings so that they can be reconstructed into a new interpretation. Deconstruction can be undertaken in a number of ways that are similar to those used in the analysis of primary qualitative studies. For example, some use a purely inductive process similar to that used in grounded theory where each study is recoded. These new codes are then examined across the studies as part of the synthesis and translation. Others begin with a list of codes already identified and against which they examine each study in isolation before progressing to synthesis. Yet others do little re-analysing of the raw data and instead focus on synthesising and translating the central concepts and metaphors identified by the author of the original study (Finfgeld, 2003). Whatever approach is chosen, the important factor is that it is transparent, justified and in keeping with the overall aim of the review. Once the individual studies are recoded the identified concepts are then juxtaposed in preparation for comparison. Constructing a grid or table of the concepts facilitates comparison but also enhances transparency.

As part of analysis and synthesis, Noblit and Hare (1988) suggest three ways in which studies can be related and translated. Reciprocal translational analysis (RTA) is the easiest or simplest form of synthesis because it involves a search for concepts and metaphors within and across studies that are similar and/or appear repeatedly (Downe, 2008). The underlying assumption of RTA is that the findings of the studies can be integrated due to their similarities (Flemming, 2007). Refutational synthesis is a search for findings of studies that refute or are in opposition to each other. This type of synthesis is valuable because it may result in the identification of another category or understanding that had not been identified in the original studies (Walsh and Downe, 2005). The third strategy is known as 'line of argument' (LOA) synthesis where the similarities and dissimilarities are examined and integrated into a new interpretation that most completely represents the emerging concepts or patterns.

All of these processes are inductive and can use strategies, such as constant comparative analysis that was originally developed for use in grounded theory but which now has wider application as a method of qualitative data analysis. In

Table 7.10 Example of Synthesis: Identity and Coping Experiences in Chronic Fatigue Syndrome

Thematic Groups from Original Studies	Second-order Analyses	Third-order Analyses
Symptom experience and consequences for everyday life	An empty battery or a blown fuse; controlled and betrayed by their bodies; bodies that no longer held the capacity for social involvement.	Identity: legitimacy of their illness being questioned; previous sense of identity became more or less invalid.
Illness beliefs and causal attributions	A classical infection striking a fragile immune system; bodily collapse due to stress and overload; definitely not a psychosomatic disorder; weak character.	Strategies for coping: knowing more about the condition; keeping a distance to protect oneself; learning to know more about their limits.
Doctor–patient interaction: 'Are you really sick?'	Negotiated the nature of the disorder; confrontations with their doctors when biomedical markers were absent; guilt, blame, shame game; challenges when a professional authority should be managed under considerable scientific uncertainty; the significance of getting a diagnosis.	

Source: L. Larun and K. Malterud, (2007) 'Identity and coping experiences in Chronic Fatigue Syndrome: a synthesis of qualitative studies', *Patient Education and Counseling*, 69: 20–8.

constant comparative analysis, one piece of data is taken and compared with all other pieces of data that are either similar or different and the outcome is theory or new knowledge. Table 7.10 presents an example of themes, second-order and third-order analyses from a synthesis of identity and coping experiences in chronic fatigue syndrome in which a meta-ethnographic approach was used (Larun and Malterud, 2007).

Some issues that require clarification have arisen around the process of synthesis in a meta-ethnography. For example, Atkins et al. (2008), in their meta-ethnography of adherence to tuberculosis treatment, identified that there was a lack of guidance in respect of how to relate and translate the concepts/metaphors from each study. Similarly, the process of synthesising translations is not clearly delineated. Decisions around these areas are complex, and considerable expertise in the areas of qualitative research, and particularly qualitative research analysis, is necessary to undertake such an endeavour. As Campbell et al. (2011) suggest, meta-ethnography should be considered an advanced qualitative research method.

Meta-study

Paterson et al. (2001) developed a meta-synthesis method derived from a general approach developed within sociology and anthropology and termed meta-study

(Thorne et al., 2002). Meta-study, as conceived by Paterson et al. (2001) aims to go beyond meta-ethnography because it examines the findings of each study (meta-data analysis), the method by which the study was conducted (meta-method) and the theory or theoretical influences underlying the study (meta-theory). This, they contend, is because research takes place in a social, historical and ideological context that affects how it is undertaken as well as shaping the results. For example, the theoretical perspective the researcher adopts has an influence on the choice of topics, the questions that are posed about those topics, the research designs that are chosen to answer those questions and the manner in which the findings are interpreted. Therefore, Paterson et al. (2001) argue, their method requires an examination of all components of the research process in order to develop a more complete interpretation and understanding of those factors that influenced the conduct and outcome of the research.

Paterson et al. (2001) separate analysis and synthesis and state that the three analytic strategies of meta-data analysis, meta-method and meta-theory must be undertaken before meta-synthesis can occur (Figure 7.2). This approach, they argue, generates new and more complete understandings of the phenomenon under study (Paterson et al., 2001: 2). See Figure 7.2 for the components of meta-study.

Meta-data analysis is the analysis of the findings of individual studies by means of processing the 'processed data' (Zhao, 1991). Processed data are the results of the analysis undertaken by the researcher. In a primary study, the researcher interprets the raw data to identify key concepts or metaphors. In meta-data analysis, it is these that form the focus of the analysis. Meta-data analysis, then, involves reinterpretation of the actual findings from the original qualitative studies in light of those from other studies (Thorne et al., 2002). The analysis proceeds by critically comparing the central concepts in each study with those in the other studies in the review for the purpose of identifying similarities and differences. Analytic methods similar to those outlined in meta-ethnography can

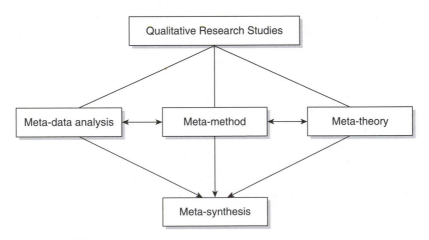

Figure 7.2   Components of Meta-study

Source: Adapted from Paterson et al. (2001)

be adopted. For example, in a meta-study of early professional socialisation and career choice in nursing, Price (2009) adopted thematic analysis as her method of data analysis.

Meta-method is an examination of the methodologies of the studies in the review. Various aspects, such as design choice, sampling, data collection and analysis, are scrutinised to determine the rigour with which the study was conducted, and the process is similar to that of critical appraisal (Barnett-Page and Thomas, 2009). However, there is an additional requirement in meta-method as conceived by Paterson et al. (2001) to determine if there was congruence between the research question and the methodology chosen to answer it. In other words, did the researcher choose the correct method to answer the question posed? In addition, the meta-synthesist should explore if the chosen methodology impacted on how the outcomes or findings of the study were conceived (Thorne et al., 2002).

Meta-theory is the examination of the philosophical and theoretical perspectives and assumptions that directed the research studies in order to determine how they might have influenced interpretation of the data. For example, in their meta-study of fatigue in chronic illness, Paterson et al. (2003) identified that most of the studies that used a phenomenological methodology focused on the phenomenon of fatigue rather than fatigue as part of the whole experience of living with a chronic illness. As a result, the findings did not consider the important social, environmental and personal factors that affected how fatigue is experienced and managed.

Meta-synthesis is undertaken when the analytic phases of meta-data analysis, meta-method and meta-theory are complete. It involves bringing together the ideas that have been taken apart and constructing a new interpretation. However, Paterson et al. (2001) give little guidance on how the three components are integrated as they were unwilling to oversimplify the process. They state that the process is non-linear and dynamic and involves thinking, interpreting, creating, theorising and reflecting.

As with meta-ethnography, meta-study is an advanced method that Paterson et al., (2001) claim should only be undertaken by seasoned researchers. To undertake such an endeavour the researcher(s) must be completely familiar with the theories and research designs that are likely to be sampled. In addition, considerable time and resources are needed to undertake the three analytical processes and subsequent synthesis. Therefore, meta-study is generally beyond the remit of undergraduate study, although the principles of the tripartite analysis of data, method and theory could be adopted and applied to any literature review. Readers requiring additional information are referred to Paterson et al.'s (2001) original text where a comprehensive account of the method is provided.

Qualitative Meta-summary

Qualitative meta-summary is a 'quantitatively oriented aggregation of qualitative findings that are themselves topical or thematic summaries or surveys of data' (Sandelowski and Barroso, 2007: 151). What this means is that a meta-summary includes a quantitative process of identifying the frequency of individual findings. It works on the assumption that qualitative and quantitative data can be transformed into one another. It differs from meta-ethnography and meta-study in that the findings of the studies are accumulated and summarised (aggregated). Sandelowski and Barroso (2003b; 2007) argue that in qualitative research some findings occur with sufficient frequency to form a pattern or theme. It is this frequency of occurrence that facilitates the quantitative transformation. They contend this gives more meaning to the extracted data and is a way of verifying the patterns and themes that emerge from the studies. Although originally developed to accommodate reports from qualitative descriptive surveys, meta-summary can also be used with the findings of quantitative descriptive studies or even syntheses of other studies (Sandelowski and Barroso, 2007; Sandelowski et al., 2007).

Box 7.5   Techniques of Qualitative Meta-summary (Adapted from Sandelowski and Barroso, 2007)

- Extracting findings.
- Editing findings.
- Grouping findings about the same topic.
- Abstracting and formatting findings.
- Calculating frequency and intensity effect sizes.

Qualitative meta-summary techniques are outlined in Box 7.5. The first step in the process is to extract findings from individual study reports or syntheses about the topic area of interest. It is important that the topic area in which the reviewer is interested is reasonably well defined. This will ensure that the appropriate findings are extracted in a consistent way. Once the findings have been extracted Sandelowski and Barroso (2007) recommend that they are edited so that they can be understood by any reader. For example, this may involve editing the themes and patterns so that they form complete sentences that are easily understood. The third technique involves grouping findings that appear to be about the same topic. For example, if the reviewer was interested in exploring the self-management practices of those who live with type II diabetes, they may identify findings from several reports that refer to dietary practices. At this point of the process these findings would be grouped together. Once all the findings have been grouped, they are abstracted. This is a process of developing statements that succinctly capture the content of all the findings and reducing them to a smaller number.

The final stage of meta-summary is determining the frequency of a finding with the assumption that the higher the frequency the greater its validity (Barnett-Page and Thomas, 2009). This is done by firstly determining the frequency effect size – that is, calculating the percentage of reports containing a particular finding against the overall number of reports. For example, if 10 reports identified that those with type II diabetes had dietary knowledge deficits and the overall number of reports was 20, then the frequency size effect would be 50 per cent (10 ÷ 20). The second part of the process is about determining the intensity size effect. Simply stated, this is about calculating the contribution of the findings in each report to the overall number of findings. For example, if an individual study contained 12 findings and the total number was 48 then the intensity size effect is 25 per cent (12 ÷ 48). Sandelowski and Barroso (2007) claim that as a result of calculating the intensity effect sizes it will be possible to see how much the findings in each study contributed overall.

Meta-summary is considered a relatively new approach but Sandelowski and Barroso (2007) claim that the technique has the potential to enhance the validity of the findings of qualitative studies, particularly in respect of the findings that have a high frequency. However, this approach is also a complex one that requires significant skills in data analysis and aggregation. Readers are referred to Sandelowski and Barroso's (2007) text for additional detail on the techniques of meta-summary.

In summary, the three approaches to meta-synthesis presented here are but a small example of a range of methods that have been and are being developed and appearing in the literature. All are complex methods that require a high level of expertise and skill in the conduct and evaluation of qualitative research. Moreover, they are limited in their applicability because they concentrate on research studies of one type or another and do not facilitate the synthesis of non-research literature. The reader is referred to Barnett-Page and Thomas (2009), Campbell et al. (2011) and Ring et al. (2011) for further detail on the range of methods being adopted for the synthesis of qualitative research.

Summary

This chapter has explored the various means by which the results of research studies can be combined and pooled. The first part of the chapter focused on the importance of presenting the results from your analysis of the literature. Examples of how the search strategy, search results, inclusion and exclusion criteria and a collation of information about each study could be presented were offered. Thematic analysis as a means of undertaking a synthesis of literature that includes research and non-research literature was presented because this is the approach you are more likely to use in literature reviews that are undertaken for an academic assignment or as a chapter in a dissertation. Additional and more complex methods of synthesis, including narrative synthesis, meta-analysis and meta-synthesis were introduced and their various techniques were presented. Although the knowledge accumulated from synthesis using these methods is key in terms of the potential impact on clinical practice and/or healthcare policy or research, they are limited in their appropriateness for the undergraduate student undertaking a literature review. Primarily, they are confined to combining research studies of one type or another and, therefore, do not facilitate the synthesis of the wide range of studies you are likely to encounter in your reading. Moreover, they do not accommodate the synthesis of non-research literature that is likely to inform, situate and contextualise your review. Nonetheless, you should now have an appreciation of the requirements of each method of synthesis, the similarities and differences between them and when each might be used.

Key Points

- Synthesis is the part of the process of the literature review where results are combined and pooled.
- In all literature reviews the first step of synthesis should be to present the findings including: the search strategy, the results of the search, inclusion and exclusion criteria and a collation of information about each study.
- Thematic analysis is most commonly undertaken in the synthesis of mixed literature – that is, research and non-research.
- Synthesis methods that are used to combine or pool the results of reviews of research studies include, but are not limited to: narrative synthesis, meta-analysis, meta-synthesis (e.g. meta-ethnography, meta-study, meta-summary).
- Narrative synthesis was developed for use where statistical analysis is not possible because of the range of different research designs included in the review. Although it can be used with mixed literature, to date its use has been primarily associated with the synthesis of multiple studies in systematic reviews.
- Meta-analysis is a process of statistical analysis of numerical data. Results are pooled and re-analysed to determine with more accuracy whether or not an intervention is effective. Studies suitable for meta-analysis must be of a similar design, with the gold standard being RCTs.
- Meta-synthesis is adopted in this text as a term that encompasses the various methods that have been developed to address the synthesis of qualitative research. Examples are meta-ethnography, meta-study and qualitative meta-summary.
- Meta-ethnography was first proposed as an alternative to meta-analysis and has emerged as the leading method for synthesis of qualitative research. Its purpose is to construct a new interpretation or theory about the phenomenon under study.
- Meta-study is an approach to synthesis that has three analytic phases. It examines the findings of each study (meta-data analysis), the method by which the study was conducted (meta-method) and the theory or theoretical influences underlying the study (meta-theory). These three analytic strategies must be undertaken before meta-synthesis can occur. The aim is to generate new and more complete understandings of the phenomenon under study.
- Qualitative meta-summary aggregates qualitative findings through a quantitative process for the purpose of determining the frequency of each finding in and across studies. It assumes that qualitative and quantitative data can be transformed into one another. It differs essentially from meta-ethnography and meta-study in that the findings are accumulated and summarised (aggregated).
- Synthesis methods are directed by the type of data (research and/or non-research literature) and the purpose of the review.

8

Writing up Your Literature Review

Introduction

Having gone through the steps of identifying a review topic, identifying and gathering the appropriate literature, organising, analysing and synthesising the literature, it is now time to consider how you will present your review to others. If your literature review is to receive appropriate recognition and add to the available knowledge on the topic being reviewed, it is essential that you present the outcomes to others both clearly and accurately, and in a manner that demonstrates your knowledge of the subject.

☑ Learning Outcomes ☑

By the end of this chapter you should be able to:

- explore how the presentation of your literature review can be structured.
- discuss some basic tips in relation to academic writing skills, grammar and syntax.

As mentioned, an important element of a good literature review is to be able to clearly and accurately disseminate your findings to others. In order to do this you have to write up your review. The structure and organisation of your review will to some degree be determined by the purpose of the review. For example, in the case of systematic reviews there are clear structures that indicate how the review should be undertaken and thus presented. However, where the review is part of a research study or is being undertaken as part of an academic programme there is usually some flexibility in relation to structuring and writing it up. However, it is expected that the review will be presented in a way that is logical and that all the key elements are included (Cronin et al., 2008).

Burns and Grove (2007) suggest that the review be structured into an introduction, followed by the main body of the literature review and ending with a conclusion. However, for stand-alone literature reviews an abstract may be required at the beginning and recommendations may be expected at the end of the review. The word count for the review and marking criteria will also influence how you structure your review.

Writing the Review

All the steps that formed your literature review need to be included as you write up your work. It is important that you are logical as to their inclusion – that is, identifying your review topic comes before your search of the literature and so forth. Many of the factors you considered when critically analysing another author's works now apply to your work. You need to reflect on your own review in the same way you considered those you reviewed for study.

ACTIVITY 8.1

Read your review when you have finished writing it up. If you were an author writing a literature review on this topic, would you have selected your review for inclusion? Why?

Title and Abstract

The title and the abstract are often the first two points of contact between you and the reader. A reader may decide to ignore or read your work based on how you have formulated your title and the information you have included in your abstract. In presenting your title and abstract first impressions are important. As a general rule your title should ideally be about 10–15 words in length. Too long and it becomes unwieldy and often confusing to the reader; too short and you may not have included sufficient information to enlighten the reader as to the intention of the review (Parahoo, 2006).

The abstract is a brief summary of your work and should contain enough details to give the reader an overall impression of what the review is about and how it was conducted. Abstracts vary in length but are usually about 150–200 words. An abstract should include some background on the problem/review topic, how the search was undertaken, including the keywords and databases used, the outcome of the review and any recommendations. Although both the title and abstract appear at the start of the review, they are usually written last.

Introduction

The purpose of the introduction is to put your literature in context. You know why you have selected this topic and why it is important, and how it can help the development of the profession; however, the reader does not necessarily know this and certainly does not understand it from your perspective. A major function of the introduction is to offer a concise background to the reader with regard to the purpose of the review. For example, you may have noticed that some post-operative patients appear to have a lot more pain than others, yet they have all had similar surgery and are receiving similar post-operative analgesia. A quick glance at some of the literature on the topic indicated there might be other reasons for the pain these patients were suffering from and so you decided to review the literature to identify these potential causes and also check how the patients might be treated or the symptoms eliminated. In this example there is the opportunity to identify the problem that 'some post-operative patients appear to have a lot more pain than others'. This can then be linked with your brief scan of the literature by citing supporting works and their suggestions that there may be other factors that exacerbate some patients' experience of pain. You are now in a position to state the purpose of your review.

The search strategy used may be identified either at the end of the introduction or at the beginning of the review of the literature section. This should include listing the keywords and keyword combinations that were used in the search, the databases and other sources that were explored and any limits that were set on the search (Cronin et al., 2008). There should be enough information included on how you conducted your search so that another reviewer could replicate the search and study selection (Bettany-Saltikov, 2012).

Although the introduction appears at the beginning of your review, it is often not finalised until the review is complete. However, having a working draft of your introduction as you conduct your review can be useful because it identifies the purpose of your review and what you are aiming to achieve. It is, therefore, important to regularly return to your introduction to ensure that you are still focused on the purpose identified.

As mentioned, the introduction is often finalised when the review is completed. At this stage the end of the review is in sight and the tendency can be to rush to get the introduction complete and wrap up this piece of work. However, the introduction is the first part of the actual literature review readers will encounter, and if you have seduced them to read further through a good title and abstract you want to continue to make a good impression. It is, therefore, worthwhile spending extra time on the introduction so as to encourage readers to read more of your work.

The Review of the Literature

This section is where the literature related to the problem or topic of interest is presented, analysed, synthesised and discussed in relation to other literature. The literature should be presented in an organised and objective manner, without personal views or opinions being expressed by the reviewer. The key research studies related to the topic being reviewed should be included in your review. The methodological approaches used in these studies should be critically analysed and the implications discussed. This analysis and its implications should be supported by reference to relevant research texts or articles. Remember, when doing this analysis, it is not a comprehensive critique that is being undertaken, but an attempt to assess the quality of the evidence being presented in the article (Polit and Beck, 2012). Nonetheless, it is important to ensure that critical details concerning the methodology of these studies or systematic reviews are included. Without these it becomes more difficult for the reader to evaluate your outcomes and recommend change (Bettany-Saltikov, 2012). Not all studies included in your review need to be critically analysed, and in some instances studies that have similar findings, or support each other, may be synopsised together (see Box 8.1).

Box 8.1   Example of Studies Summarised Together

... in the USA, the level of anxiety of nursing students about caring for people with HIV/AIDS was reduced by education (All & Sullivan 1997). This view was shared in Singapore, where Ngan et al. (2000, p. 32) found that 'weaknesses in the provision of education must be addressed'. These findings are supported by studies conducted in Turkey (Bektas & Kulakac 2007), South Africa (Madumo & Peu 2006), Germany (Lohrmann et al., 2000) and Jordan (Petro-Nustas et al., 2002).

(Pickles et al., 2009: 2265)

Studies and works that have similar themes are usually arranged under sub-headings. These studies are then analysed, discussed and synthesised in an attempt to identify new meanings or ideas. When writing your review, you should interpret and paraphrase the information gleaned from the literature. Threading together a series of passages or quotations from different studies without undertaking analyses or interpretation usually indicates a failure to internalise and comprehend the significance of that literature, and often results in students losing crucial marks in their literature review.

When reading studies to include in your literature review you will have noticed that some of the studies can be cited under more than one sub-heading. If a study is included under a number of sub-headings it only needs to be critically reviewed once; it is not necessary to reanalyse the study under subsequent headings. When presenting literature with similar themes, the characteristic that connects or differentiates these studies is the findings. It is, therefore, important to present the findings early when discussing a study. In doing this, it is also crucial to ensure that the studies and their findings match the theme of the sub-heading under which they are being included.

When examining the literature in your review, not all the studies or authors you will encounter will have the same perspective or views. Some may have findings or opinions that are at variance with commonly held views. It is important when presenting your review that recognition is given to alternative findings and theories; you are not saying they are correct, but you are acknowledging they exist. It can also be useful to compare studies that have very different findings. Were there differences in the way the studies were undertaken that might have led to these atypical outcomes?

Was there a difference in how the samples were selected, or the size of the samples for example?

When writing your review it is important to remember that quantitative research is mainly built on probability; nothing is definitive but perhaps is likely to be the case. It is similar to a famous lager that does not claim to be the best lager in the world; it only 'probably' is. Qualitative research is based on the views and perspectives of individuals and does not claim generalisablity to the population. So when you are writing your review it is important to avoid words that generalise or are definitive when describing the findings of a study. Statements to avoid include 'it is obvious that ...' and 'it is evident ...'. More appropriate statements would be 'it appears that...' and 'it seems ...'. The latter statements indicate what appears to be, but also allow for the element of chance, which in some instances does play a role.

It is important to remember that a review is more than simply descriptive. The role of the reviewer is to analyse the literature in order to evaluate the data, compare the literature for similarities and differences, and to identify plausible rationales for any inconsistencies that may exist (Polit and Beck, 2012).

Conclusion

The conclusion is a succinct overview of the salient points within the literature review and the deductions and possible outcomes that the reviewer has established while analysing and synthesising the literature. Reviewers often commence the conclusion by restating the review question or problem. This is followed by a short summary of what is known about the topic, areas where there is a dearth of information or deficit in the knowledge base, and the identification of inconsistencies in the literature. Arguments central to the review are presented in a concise manner and, finally, conclusions are identified. Again it is important that these conclusions correspond with the initial review problem.

This is the part of the review where you, the reviewer, have an opportunity to objectively put forward your opinions. However, this is not a *carte blanche* to say whatever you want. Your comments need to be supported by the literature, be objectively presented, and relate to the analysis and synthesis you have done.

The conclusion to a large degree summarises your review. No new studies or information should, therefore, be presented at this stage. If a piece of evidence is important enough to be included here, then it should have been in the main body of the review.

Recommendations

Having completed the review and identified your conclusions, what do you feel should happen next? Recommendations are an opportunity for you, the reviewer, to suggest the next steps for the reader. Those steps should be consistent with your conclusions, and may suggest a change of practice or that the information available is inconclusive and that practice should remain the same for the present. As a result of inconsistencies between studies, perhaps you believe that more research is needed into this topic. If so, it is better to be specific and identify the purpose of research you are recommending (Whittaker and Williamson, 2011). Recommendations may be part of the conclusion or a separate heading; this depends on the presentation and marking guidelines for the review.

References

At the end of your literature review there should be a full bibliographical reference list of all source material contained therein. All of the journal articles, books and other media that were cited in your review need to be included in your reference list. Failing to acknowledge another author's work can lead to claims of plagiarism, which is regarded as a serious offence (see Chapter 9 for more information on referencing and plagiarism).

Writing, Grammar and Syntax

When writing your review it is important to check if there are any academic conventions you need to adhere to. Academic conventions can include the method of referencing you are expected to use (see Chapter 9), the layout of your review and the use of the third person. In the latter case there is some debate within academic writing circles as to whether it is appropriate to use 'I' in a sentence or to refer to yourself as 'the author' or 'the reviewer'. The use of the third person, in some instances, is seen as more objective, but Aveyard (2010) adds that it can also be a source of confusion, leaving the reader unsure to whom the writer of the review is referring. It is a good idea, if you are using the third person to refer to yourself, to pick one title that you use throughout your work. Constantly changing between 'this author', 'writer' or 'reviewer' will potentially lead to confusion. Again, it is important to check if there are academic conventions that you are expected to adhere to and to follow them, as failure to do so can lead to a loss of marks.

When writing your review it is important to do so correctly. You should use proper sentences. A sentence starts with a capital letter, it should contain a subject, a verb and an object, and it ends with a full stop. While this seems basic, it is not unusual for full stops, capital letters and other parts of sentences to be omitted. The result is usually a lack of clarity as to what the writer is attempting to communicate. Keep your sentences simple and focus on one concept. Keep your sentences short, a maximum of 14 to 16 words, unless you are good at punctuation. Otherwise there is a likelihood the reader will end up reading the sentence a number of times to try to make sense of it. Ensure that your sentences have a logical flow and that they link with the preceding sentences.

It is a good idea to link your paragraphs. This can be done by finishing a paragraph with a sentence identifying the content in the next section. Introduce the main theme when starting a new paragraph and ensure that the theme is maintained throughout the paragraph (Bettany-Saltikov, 2012). By doing this you should have a logical flow within both your sentences and paragraphs and thus within your review.

Paragraphs should have more than one sentence. A common error is to hit the return key instead of the spacebar, and the result is a new paragraph. One-sentence paragraphs usually lack continuity and undermine the flow of your work.

Other considerations are spelling and grammar. UK spelling of some words differs from US spelling – for example, oesophagus (esophagus) and theatre (theater) – so it is important to use the conventions of the country in which you are studying. If you are using a spell check on your computer, make sure it is set to the relevant version of English. Ensure that sentences are complete and that words have not been omitted. It is important to include both the definite article (the) and the indefinite article (a) as appropriate. The proper use of punctuation can make reading a literature review so much simpler. Conversely, poor punctuation can totally change the meaning of a sentence and cause confusion for the reader. Computer spelling and grammar checks can be set to help with punctuation, but it is useful to know a little about it. There are texts available that are amusing yet helpful in coming to terms with English grammar and punctuation, such as *Eats, Shoots & Leaves* (Truss, 2003).

Consistency in the use of tenses is important. The majority of the main body of the literature review will be in the past tense as it will consist of the presentation and appraisal of studies that have already been undertaken. However, other sections, such as identifying the purpose, will be written in the present tense. It is important to use tenses appropriately and to maintain the same tense within a sentence and ideally within a paragraph.

Jargon should be avoided, and if a particular slang term needs to be used it should be placed in inverted commas. 'Texting' language should not be used when writing your literature review. Indeed, any form of abbreviation should be used with caution, and only recognised abbreviations used. When using acronyms use the full form in the first instance with the abbreviated form beside it in brackets, for example Department of Health (DoH). After this the acronym DoH can be used.

It is always a good idea to get someone to read your review before you submit the final work. During the course of completing the review you can become so familiar with what you are writing that typing mistakes, such as omitted words or wrong tenses, can be missed. Ensure the individual you ask to read your work is someone who will give you critical feedback, not someone who will tell you it is great just to keep you happy.

Undertaking and writing your review is a time-consuming endeavour and many students and novice reviewers underestimate how long it takes. It is important to give sufficient time to all aspects of the review as writing up your review is, in its own way, as important as identifying the review topic and searching the literature. The former will highlight the efforts made in undertaking the review, and will become the evidence by which your literature review will be evaluated.

Summary

Having undertaken the steps of the review process it is now necessary that you describe to the reader how you completed these steps, and discuss the decisions that were made in searching and selecting the literature, and how the analysis and synthesis of this literature were undertaken. This written record will be the evidence on which your review will be judged, and it needs to be presented clearly, accurately and with attention to detail. In writing up your review it is important to follow a logical sequence, beginning with why you selected this topic for your review through to your summary and recommendations. Good grammar and syntax (sentence structure) play an important part in indicating attention to detail. So create a good first impression.

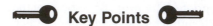 **Key Points**

- Your literature review will be judged on the evidence supplied by you in the written presentation – so accuracy, clarity and attention to detail are very important.
- There should be a logical consistency to how your review is presented.
- Good grammar and proper syntax are important elements of good writing.
- Remember, first impressions count.

9

Referencing and Plagiarism

Introduction

Accurate referencing is important when undertaking a literature review or indeed any form of academic writing. Referencing serves a number of important functions: it can be used to support assertions and comments made by the reviewer; it is used to acknowledge the work of other authors; and it allows the reader the opportunity to access the primary works cited by the reviewer (Davids et al., 2010). Poor adherence to referencing conventions increases the risk that elements of the work may be regarded as being plagiarised. The purpose of this chapter is to offer some guidance on referencing, both in the text and in the bibliographical reference section at the end of a literature review. This chapter will also focus on how accidental plagiarism can be avoided through the use of good referencing techniques.

☑ Learning Outcomes ☑

By the end of this chapter you should be able to:

- Reference literature in the text of your review.
- Complete a bibliographical reference section at the end of your review.
- Describe what plagiarism is.
- Use good referencing techniques to avoid accidental plagiarism.

Referencing

In all forms of communication, but particularly in academic writing, it is important to acknowledge the work of other authors who are quoted directly or whose work is paraphrased. Failing to do this can be regarded as academic fraud or plagiarism. There are two places within a literature review where referencing is required. They are in the text where the cited work is presented and at the end of the work in the bibliographical reference section (Ridley, 2008).

Referencing, as stated earlier, has a number of important roles within academic writing, some of which can be seen in Box 9.1. In your literature review you will be presenting the works of many different authors. In presenting these studies the authors' names and the dates of publications (or a citation number in the case of the Vancouver system) becomes the in-text method of identifying individual works to the reader. It is, therefore, important to accurately reference that work so the reader can clearly identify it. Some common errors that occur are often attributed to non-attention to detail where the reviewer uses a wrong date, or includes or excludes other authors (et al.) either of which changes the unique identifier and implies this is a different piece of work.

Box 9.1   Purposes of Referencing

- Provides a unique identifier for each work presented within the review.
- Supports assertions and comments made in the review.
- Acknowledges the works of other authors.
- Demonstrates how widely you have read on and around the topic.
- Allows the reader to access the original works presented within the review.

In reviewing the literature it is important to remain objective and report both sides of a debate. Sometimes it is necessary to report assertions that you, the reviewer, do not agree with or that have later been reported as incorrect. Excluding such information can weaken an argument considerably; however, novice reviewers may feel reluctant to include this information for fear that it may be attributed to them. Conversely, good referencing can demonstrate that this is clearly not the case. Similarly, the reviewer should also strive to ensure that all authors' works are correctly and accurately acknowledged.

As stated earlier, it is important to acknowledge the original author of any piece of work, whether it is published or unpublished. It is important to do this to avoid plagiarism but also to give recognition to the work of others. Citation indices record how frequently authors are cited by their peers in other publications and offer a form of analysis in relation to the impact of the work. Journals are also ranked by these indices. The more frequently articles from a particular journal are cited, the higher its impact factor. The impact of an article or where it is published can have an effect on how that work is viewed by peers, and so it is important to give recognition to the original author.

ACTIVITY 9.1

Consider the Following Scenario

After expending considerable time and energy undertaking your literature review, and preparing it for and getting it published, you find a large portion of it used in another article without any acknowledgement that this is your work. How would you feel, as it now appears that this author is claiming your work as their own?

Alternatively, the reviewer did acknowledge the work, but cited another person as the author – not you. So now someone else is receiving academic recognition for your work. Would you be happy?

Citing Other Authors

The two ways of citing the work of other authors in your review are: directly quoting the original text, or paraphrasing the information you wish to convey. Quotation is taking a section of the original work and presenting it word for word within your literature review. Quotations are usually identified by placing the quoted section in inverted commas or as an indented block that is single-line spaced. The former is usually used for short quotations whereas the latter is used for a long quotation. The author, the year of publication and the page number of the book or article where the quotation appears also need to be included in the in-text reference. Examples of both types of quotation can be seen in Box 9.2.

Box 9.2   Quotations

Use of Inverted Commas

On the subject of referencing Cronin et al. (2008: 43) state that 'Regardless of whether the review is part of a course of study or for publication, it is an essential part of the process that all sourced material is acknowledged.' They continue by stating that ...

Block quotation

Cronin et al. state that all material cited should be referenced and identify some of consequences of not adhering to good referencing techniques.

> Regardless of whether the review is part of a course of study or for publication, it is an essential part of the process that all sourced material is acknowledged. This means that every citation in the text must appear in the reference/ bibliography and vice versa. Omissions or errors in referencing are very common and students often lose vital marks in assignment [sic] because of it.

(Cronin et al., 2008: 43)

As stated earlier, quotations should appear exactly as they appear in the original text. Grammatical or spelling errors should not be corrected. If an error is identified, the Latin word *sic* (*sic erat scriptum* – thus it was written) is usually placed in square brackets after the error – for example, 'I know you herd [sic] what I said.'

It is important not to overuse quotations when undertaking a literature review or any form of academic writing. Quotations should be used sparingly and are best used to emphasise rather than explain a point. Excessive use of quotations often appears like a mosaic of other authors' ideas and suggests a lack of contextual understanding on the part of the reviewer (Ridley, 2008). Quotations, when used, should maintain the continuity of the sentence or paragraph within which they occur. All too frequently, students and novice writers include a quotation that is outside the natural flow of the sentence. This is sometimes because the quoted sentence does not fit in its complete state within the reviewer's sentence. One way of overcoming this is to omit part of the quotation. This is usually indicated by the inclusion of an ellipsis (…) to indicate something has been omitted. However, in doing this, the reviewer must ensure they are not changing the meaning of what was written (Box 9.3).

Box 9.3   Using an Ellipsis

Cronin et al. (2008: 43) state that '… every citation in the text must appear in the reference/bibliography and vice versa'.

The most common method of presenting another author's work is paraphrasing. Paraphrasing involves presenting an author's ideas or findings in your own words. However, the original authors must be acknowledged by having their names and the year of publication identified, either as part of the sentence or at the end of the paraphrase. It is not usually necessary to include a page number in the text when paraphrasing; however, it is not incorrect to do so. An example of both of these methods of paraphrasing can be seen in Box 9.4.

Box 9.4   Paraphrasing

Example 1

Cronin et al. (2008) state that works by other authors must be acknowledged, both in the text and in the reference/bibliography at the end of the work. Errors in referencing are common and can result in students receiving poorer marks for submitted work.

Example 2

All works by other authors that the reviewer refers to must be acknowledged in the text and in the reference/bibliography section. Poor referencing occurs frequently and can lead to a student receiving a poorer grade in an assignment (Cronin et al., 2008).

Another purpose of referencing is to demonstrate how widely you have read around a topic. It is important in a literature review to show you have read widely on the topic and that the most significant works have been included in your review. Word limits may restrict the number of articles that you will be able to review. However, it will always be a balancing act between being too broad (including too many articles and not analysing them adequately) and being too in-depth (offering a comprehensive analysis on a limited number of articles). Academic assignment guidelines may address this by suggesting a minimum number of references, so it is important to read these guidelines carefully.

Finally, references allow the reader to access the original works that are included in your literature review. There are a number of reasons why readers may wish to do this, including to source articles for their own assignments or reviews, to gain a greater insight into a particular issue discussed within the review, to check the accuracy of interpretations made within the review, or simply to check if those references are accurate or exist. It is, therefore, important to ensure that the references in the text and the references at the end of the review are accurate and do match.

Readers will naturally move from the citation in the text to the bibliographical reference at the end of the review if they are accessing articles. Common referencing errors that occur here are that:

- the date of publication of the citation and reference do not match
- 'et al.' is omitted or is incorrectly included in the citation
- the full bibliographical reference is not included.

In the first two cases the reader does not know if the difference is due to lack of attention to detail, is a different article that is being referred to, or which reference, if either, is correct. In the latter case the reader has no reference to access. Poor referencing undermines the integrity of your review and can lead to a poorer mark being received for the work (Cronin et al., 2008). It is, therefore, worth investing time to ensure that references are accurate and complete.

Plagiarism

Plagiarism is regarded as a form of academic fraud and involves presenting the work of another author without due recognition or acknowledgement. In this situation the writer appears to be claiming someone else's work as their own. Zafron (2012) states that students often fail to realise that not giving due recognition to another's work, when quoting or paraphrasing, constitutes plagiarism. Most third-level institutions regard plagiarism as a serious offence and can impose strong sanctions on anyone who is deemed to have plagiarised. Ignorance of plagiarism is rarely accepted as an excuse as it is the action rather than the intent that is penalised. Therefore, whether your review is an academic submission or for publication, due recognition must be given to the original authors of cited works.

Plagiarism does not simply apply to another author's work, it also applies to previous work undertaken by a writer that was published or submitted for an academic assignment. It is regarded as plagiarism to attempt to get the same piece of work published in more than one journal. Generally, third-level institutions will not accept work that was previously submitted on another course or for another assignment. Finally, if you are using your own published work in a review you must cite yourself.

With the increase in technology and wide access to obscure journals and books it may seem that plagiarism would be difficult to identify. However, differences in writing styles and in how ideas are presented from one part of a literature review to another will draw the attention of an experienced reader. Technology also helps identify plagiarism with tools such as *Turnitin* and *Safe Assignment*, which compare submissions to published and other students' works to identify similarities.

Avoiding Plagiarism

Plagiarism often occurs when students unknowingly or unwittingly fail to acknowledge another author's contribution. However, a study by Walker (2010) suggests that a small number of students knowingly indulge in plagiarism. Walker (2010) offers three different examples of plagiarism:

- *Sham paraphrasing:* This involves the use of direct quotations without indenting or using quotation marks. The material is cited as if the writer had paraphrased the original work rather than just directly transcribed it.
- *Verbatim:* This is similar to sham paraphrasing except the writer does not cite the original source and thus claims authorship of the transcribed material.
- *Purloining:* In this case the writer submits, as their own, work that has either extensively or entirely been done by another individual. There is usually some attempt to paraphrase but no recognition is given to the original author.

It is important to read all the writing guidelines that are linked to your course and assignment as plagiarism will usually be discussed within these. When preparing your notes from articles and books it is important to accurately record the bibliographical reference for those sources so that you can add both the in-text and bibliographical reference. When making notes it is important to differentiate between quotations and what you have paraphrased. Zafron (2012) identifies the art of copying and pasting as one that can lead to plagiarism difficulties for students. Often students copy and paste with the intention of reviewing a section later, but then due to time constraints or poor management of notes this literature gets included as a student's own work (Zafron, 2012).

Before you submit your review, it is important to read through your work and check each citation carefully with the appropriate reference to ensure that they match and that the reference is accurate. Referencing demands time and patience if it is to be done correctly. Tools like *Turnitin* and *Safe Assignment* can also be used to check your work to see if there are any cases of inadvertent plagiarism. However, these tools will not identify missing or inaccurate references or citations.

Referencing/Citation Conventions

There are a number of different referencing/citation conventions, and factors such as professional, institutional or publisher preference often determine which convention is used. The overview of the conventions presented here are common variations of these conventions, so in all cases it is recommended that you check and use the recommended guidelines for your course or assignment. An important consideration, no matter which system you are using, is consistency. It is important to keep the same format for all journals, books and other material you cite throughout your work and include in your references. 'References' occur at the end of your literature review and are a list of the citations that you presented in your review. A 'bibliography' is a reading list – a catalogue of the books and articles you read to inform yourself about the subject, but which might not be included in your references. It, also, is situated at the end of a review. In some instances, the terms 'references' and 'bibliography' are used interchangeably; however, technically there is a difference between these two lists. Depending on your guidelines you may not have to include a bibliography, but you will have to include a set of references.

Harvard

The Harvard referencing system is one of the most commonly used conventions within academic circles. It is a broad designation that encompasses all styles that use the author–date system of in-text referencing (University of Queensland Library, 2012). Therefore, while the basic principles are common to all Harvard referencing systems, there are also some variations within these. The main area in which variations occur is in the use of punctuation. It is, therefore, important to be familiar with how punctuation is applied within the system you are using. In the Harvard system the bibliographical references at the end are known as a Reference List and are presented in alphabetical order starting with the author's surname. Full bibliographical references, including the names of all the authors, must be included. In the text, if an article or a book has more than two authors 'et al.' is placed after the first author to identify that there are other authors. Examples of a reference list for books and journals, and of in-text referencing are presented in Box 9.5.

Box 9.5   Example of a Harvard Referencing List and In-text Referencing

Reference List

Cronin, P., Ryan, F. and Coughlan, M. (2008) 'Undertaking a literature review: a step-by-step approach', *British Journal of Nursing*, 17 (1): 38–43.

Rebar, C.R., Gersch, C.J., MacNee, C.L. and McCabe, S. (2011) *Understanding Nursing Research*. 3rd ed. Philadelphia: Wolters Kluwer/Lippincott Williams & Wilkins.

Ridley, D. (2008) *The Literature Review: A Step-by-Step Guide for Students*. London: Sage Publications Ltd.

Walker, J. (2010) 'Measuring plagiarism: researching what students do, not what they say they do', *Studies in Higher Education*, 35 (1): 41–59.

In Text

Cronin et al. (2008) state that works ...

Poor referencing occurs frequently and can lead to a student receiving a poorer grade in an assignment (Cronin et al., 2008)

American Psychological Association (APA)

APA referencing is similar to the Harvard system in that is a variation of the author–date in-text referencing system. As a result, there are some similarities between these referencing styles but also some differences. Some institutions use a Harvard/APA system for referencing. The APA system is frequently the convention of choice within the social sciences. In-text referencing is similar to Harvard's. The bibliographical references at the end are known as references and, as in the Harvard system, are presented in alphabetical order. An example of an APA references list for books and journals, and in-text referencing are presented in Box 9.6.

Box 9.6   Example of APA References

References

Cronin, P., Ryan, F., & Coughlan, M. (2008). Undertaking a literature review: a step-by-step approach. *British Journal of Nursing*, 17(1), 38–43.

Rebar, C.R., Gersch, C.J., MacNee, C.L., & McCabe, S. (2011). *Understanding nursing research* (3rd ed.). Philadelphia: Wolters Kluwer/Lippincott Williams & Wilkins.

Ridley, D. (2008). *The literature review: a step-by-step guide for students*. London: Sage Publications Ltd.

Walker, J. (2010). Measuring plagiarism: researching what students do, not what they say they do. *Studies in Higher Education*, 35(1), 41–59.

In Text

Cronin et al. (2008) state that works …

Poor referencing occurs frequently and can lead to a student receiving a poorer grade in an assignment (Cronin et al. 2008).

Vancouver

The Vancouver referencing system is, like the Harvard system, a broad designation that encompasses all systems that use a number-based, in-text referencing system (University of Queensland Library, 2012). This system uses a number in the text instead of an author and date. The first reference is numbered (1) and so on, and the reference section is presented in numerical order with (1) being the first reference. Each time that a reference is made the allocated citation number appears in the text. In both books and journals the date appears at the end of the reference. The title of the journal appears in the Medline abbreviated form and is followed by a full stop. Examples of Vancouver references for books and journals, and in-text referencing are presented in Box 9.7.

Box 9.7   Example of Vancouver References

References

1   Ridley D. The literature review: a step-by-step guide for students. London: Sage Publications Ltd; 2008.

2   Walker J. Measuring plagiarism: researching what students do, not what they say they do. Stud High Educ 2010; 35(1), 41–59.
3   Rebar CR, Gersch CJ, MacNee CL, McCabe S. Understanding nursing research. (3rd ed.). Philadelphia: Wolters Kluwer/Lippincott Williams & Wilkins: 2011.
4   Cronin P, Ryan F, Coughlan M. Undertaking a literature review: a step-by-step approach. Br J Nurs 2008; 17(1), 38–43.

In Text

Cronin et al. (4) state that works …

Poor referencing occurs frequently and can lead to a student receiving a poorer grade in an assignment (4).

There are other referencing conventions and styles, such as the use of footnotes and endnotes. However, these are generally specific requirements within courses or disciplines and as such will not be discussed here.

Summary

The aim of this chapter was to highlight the importance of good referencing. Good referencing can help support a writer's assertions, can offer the reader the opportunity to delve further into the topic, and acknowledges the work of other authors. The use of a good referencing technique reduces the likelihood that a writer will accidentally fail to acknowledge another author's work and risk being accused of plagiarism. There are a number of different conventions that offer guidance regarding how to present references. However, it is important to follow the conventions that are identified for your assignment or in your college handbook. If no conventions are recommended then remember to be consistent within the style that you select.

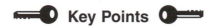 **Key Points**

- Accurate referencing is an essential part of a literature review.
- Failure to reference another author's work may be regarded as plagiarism, a form of academic fraud.
- To avoid plagiarism, ensure all media information that is quoted or paraphrased within your review is accurately referenced, both in the text and in the reference section at the end.
- When referencing, be consistent and follow the conventions that are recommended for your literature review or course.

Further Information

Anglia Ruskin University: Harvard system
http://libweb.anglia.ac.uk/referencing/harvard.htm

Cardiff University: Reference guides, tutorials and podcasts
www.cardiff.ac.ukinsrv/educationandtraining/guides/citingreferences/index.html

University of Cambridge: Referencing convention guidelines and tutorials
www.admin.cam.ac.uk/univ/plagiarism/students/referencing/conventions.html

University of Leicester: Avoiding plagiarism
www2.le.ac.uk/offices/careers/ld/resources/study/avoiding-plagiarism

University of Leicester: Referencing and bibliographies
www2.le.ac.uk/offices/careers/ld/resources/writing/writing-resources/ref-bib/

University of Leicester: Vancouver (numbered) system
www2.le.ac.uk/library/help/citing/vancouver-numbered-system/vancouver-numbered-system

University of Queensland: Referencing styles
www.library.uq.edu.au/infoskil/styles2.html

10

What Comes Next?

Introduction

The final chapter of this book is a brief outline of what you might do when you have finished your literature review. As has been indicated throughout this book, there are many reasons for undertaking a literature review and, to a large degree, this will determine what you do next. In the chapter on systematic reviews it was suggested that a plan for disseminating the findings is developed at the protocol stage, with the intention of ensuring that the outcomes reach the intended audience, be they practitioners, end-users, policy makers, organisations or commissioners of research. Inherent in this is the belief that without dissemination the findings are rendered valueless. This does not only apply to systematic reviews. Reviews that form part of a dissertation or have been written for the primary purpose of an academic assignment have the potential to be published in one form or another. This chapter focuses on some avenues for dissemination of these types of literature review. For detailed consideration of the dissemination of the results of systematic reviews the reader is referred to CRD (2009), Bettany-Saltikov (2012) and Gough et al. (2012).

☑ **Learning Outcomes** ☑

By the end of this chapter you should be able to:

- identify possible avenues for the dissemination of the findings of your literature review.
- outline the issues involved in submitting a literature review for publication in a journal.
- explain how a literature review can be submitted for a verbal presentation or poster at a conference, seminar or workshop.

For most of us who have undertaken a narrative review as part of an academic assignment, the goal is to successfully complete the assessment and we give little consideration to doing anything else with it. Similarly, although we prepare a plan for dissemination of research findings when we conduct a study as part of an academic award, we do not often consider publishing the literature review chapter. Yet a well-conducted literature review may produce findings that are of interest to your discipline and it is worth considering how you might share them.

Much of the literature that addresses dissemination tends to focus on means of sharing the results of research studies or systematic reviews. However, some of these can also be used and applied to various types of literature review. Broadly, these can include a written report that is published as an article in an academic or professional journal, a verbal report or poster at a conference, seminar or workshop, or even a journal club (Gerrish and Lacey, 2010).

Writing an Article for a Journal

Writing an article for publication in a journal has been the most widely used means of dissemination and it is likely to reach the widest audience, both nationally and internationally. This is because many journals are now available online or through open access, and accessibility has been greatly enhanced. However, for a novice, preparing an article for submission to a journal can be an overwhelming prospect and many may consider their work is not of a publishable standard. Nonetheless, those who do make the effort have the potential, at the very least, to raise awareness or provoke discussion about the topic in question that may identify, for example, implications for future practice, education and research in the area.

For a person new to publication, it is suggested that co-authoring with another who has published previously is beneficial. Although the choice of co-author is a personal one, it is worth considering the person who originally suggested the work could be published. It is a good idea at the beginning of the process that you establish how you will work together and the role and contribution each will make to the overall preparation and submission. Most journal articles now ask for a declaration that each author contributed to the preparation of the article. It is not sufficient that a person's name is included simply because they were a tutor or supervisor. Moreover, as the work belongs to you, first authorship should remain with you.

Choosing a journal for publication is an important step and requires careful consideration. It is probably worth discussing with your co-author the message you wish to convey and to what readership. Price (2010) suggests that an article can be written for a number of purposes, some of which may be applicable to your literature review. For example, your review findings may indicate that ways of looking at a topic need to be challenged or reconsidered. In terms of readership, some journals have a more academic, advanced practitioner or postgraduate readership whilst others are directed more towards practising professionals with a particular emphasis on clinical issues. It is important that you determine at the outset how your proposed article would fit with the overall ethos of the journal. The overwhelming majority have dedicated websites that can tell you about the journal, its focus and the types of article it publishes.

One thing you should be able to discern from the journal website is where it is published, which will give you a sense of its international reach. While it is not suggested that journals do not publish international work, the focus of some topics might have a more national than international appeal and are therefore more suited for publication in the jurisdiction in which the journal is published. An example of this is Jones' (2005) critical review of the literature on the evaluation of pressure ulcer prevention devices published in the UK-based *Journal of Wound Care*. The review identifies the controversy that exists about what pressure ulcer devices are most clinically efficacious and cost effective. Whilst this problem is very likely to be relevant in other healthcare jurisdictions, the problem, solutions and outcomes of the review are contextualised to the UK National Health Service, which reduces its applicability to other settings. Therefore, if Jones wished to publish the review in the American-based *Journal of Wound, Ostomy and Continence Nursing*, the problem would have had to be constructed to suit a more international readership.

Another issue that can be determined from accessing journal websites is the type of journal article that the editorial board seeks to publish. This is extremely important in terms of successfully publishing your work. Whilst most journals accommodate the publication of literature reviews, some have specific criteria for publication that may be beyond what was achieved in a traditional or narrative review. For example, the websites for journals such as *Physiotherapy* and the *Journal of Advanced Nursing* (JAN) indicate a preference for various types of protocol-driven reviews such as qualitative, quantitative and mixed-method systematic reviews, systematic methodological, economic and policy reviews, realist and integrative reviews. Conversely, other journals such as *Nursing Standard* and the *British Journal of Nursing* do not specify the type of literature review they accept. This means that if you have conducted a thorough and comprehensive traditional or narrative review on a particular aspect of nursing it will be considered for publication. These differences in publication criteria largely reflect the variation in the intended purpose of different journals and the readership to which they are directed.

A further strategy in the process of determining the journal to which you wish to submit is to read back issues. Reading previously published literature review articles will not only assist with the types of reviews that are published but may help you to understand more fully the submission guidelines for structuring the manuscript.

Once you have decided on which journal to pursue, you should access the author guidelines on the journal website. Although you may have structured your original review differently, it is crucial that you follow these guidelines closely. Failure to do so delays the review process at best and at worst can result in a rejection of your article. A key part of revising and preparing your literature review for submission is ensuring that you seek feedback on your drafts. A more experienced co-author can be very helpful at this stage by providing feedback and suggestions about how the article can be developed. Even if you have chosen to publish alone, it is still advisable to seek feedback from peers or colleagues who can provide advice on how to improve the paper. Before you submit your article you should ensure that you have met the manuscript preparation criteria specified by the journal, such as font size, formatting, submitting figures and tables and use of the preferred referencing system. Particular attention should be paid to ensuring that you have included all the references you have cited.

The majority of journals now require electronic submission through a manuscript tracking system. This has the advantage of giving instant feedback on the submission process and allows you to track the progress of your article by providing you with a unique code. Although completing the submission process can take some time, most allow you to save what you have done and return to it later. Manuscript tracking systems also permit you to review the document before final submission. Once completed, it is usual to receive a confirmation email.

The journal's website should provide you with information regarding the review process. Many journals undertake what is known as an editorial review before sending the manuscript to independent reviewers. The purpose of this is to make an initial assessment of the suitability of the article. This process also facilitates prompt feedback to the author. In the event of a paper being rejected it enables earlier submission to an alternative journal. If it is deemed an appropriate publication it is subjected to a blind peer review by at least two reviewers. You may be asked, as part of the submission process, to suggest a possible reviewer but in other instances journals retain a list of reviewers who have expertise in a particular area. Reviewers are asked to appraise submissions against specified criteria that are usually associated with the relevance of the topic to the discipline and the readership. In terms of rigour, reviewers are asked to provide feedback on the comprehensiveness of the review and its potential contribution to practice and/or knowledge. Other aspects that are considered are writing style and the clarity with which the content of the review is presented. This process can take some time, ranging from weeks to months.

Once the review process has been completed, the author receives the reviewer feedback and an editorial decision regarding publication. A paper may be accepted but with requests for revision that can range from major to minor. In this situation, the author is usually given a time limit for resubmission with amendments. Although revisions can necessitate substantial additional work it is worth completing them and attending to the reviewers' comments as you will then have the satisfaction of having your paper published. If major revisions are required, the paper may be sent for a second review.

It may also happen that your paper is rejected. Despite the fact that most people who publish will have experienced this, the first time it happens is quite disappointing and frustrating. Although it feels like a comment on the quality of your work, it may be that the topic is not consistent with the current focus of the journal. It is important, therefore, to attend carefully to the reviewers' comments as they often suggest how the paper might be developed for publication in an alternative journal.

Once revisions have been completed and approved, you will receive notification of the acceptance of your paper. Prior to publication, you will receive proofs of the article to check. You may be asked also for clarification and/or to correct any mistakes or omissions. It is very important that you check the proofs carefully as editorial changes may have been made to the original paper. At this juncture, you should make sure that you are satisfied that any changes that have been made do not distort the intended message. If you are dissatisfied with the changes, you must inform the editor.

From the first submission of an article to publication can take many months, which to some extent is dictated by the review and revision processes. However, many journals now publish online ahead of paper publication and this has shortened the process.

Preparing a Verbal Presentation

Presenting a paper is another method of disseminating the findings of your literature review, and the process is considerably quicker than publishing a journal article.

Papers can be presented in a number of settings, such as conferences, seminars, workshops and journal clubs.

The principles for choosing where you wish to present are very similar to those for deciding on an appropriate journal for an article. Primarily, you should focus on the purpose of your presentation and the audience to whom you wish to disseminate the findings of your literature review.

Presenting a paper at a conference is a popular means of sharing findings. There are numerous local, national and international conferences held every year and choosing the most appropriate one at which to present can be a daunting task. It is, therefore, advisable to consult with an experienced colleague to help you make the decision about which conference to target. Academics, senior practitioners or managers may be more familiar with potentially suitable conferences. Moreover, most conferences focus on a theme such as practice, education, research or management and it is important that your paper addresses this.

When the idea for presenting at a conference is first mooted you may feel anxious or nervous about presenting your work in a public setting. This is particularly the case when it is your first time, and it may influence your decision about whether to present locally, nationally or internationally. Many health service providers host annual conferences and you may feel more comfortable presenting locally to a familiar audience. Alternatively, some universities host student conferences that provide the opportunity to showcase students' work within a less perturbing environment. A further option is to consider seminars or workshops, which often focus on areas of specialist practice.

Regardless of which setting you ultimately choose, it is likely that you will be required to submit an abstract for review to the organisers. An abstract is essentially a summary of the paper you wish to present and it is the only means by which the selection panel can decide whether or not to accept your submission. Therefore, the golden rule for preparing an abstract is to follow the conference/seminar/workshop guidelines very closely. In addition, the abstract may subsequently appear in a book of abstracts that enables conference delegates to decide which presentations they wish to attend. Therefore, it is important that it is clear, succinct and accurate.

Following review by the selection panel you will be informed if your abstract has been accepted. It is at this time that you can begin to plan how you will deliver your paper. For most, the presentation time is between 20 and 30 minutes with 5 to 10 minutes for a question-and-answer session. Your paper is likely to be part of a concurrent session where other presentations around a generally similar topic area are presented alongside yours. Adherence to the time allocated is, therefore, fundamental to the smooth running of the session and should be a key factor when preparing your presentation.

Keeping to a strict time allocation is a difficult task. Many speakers want to present as much of their material they can. For the most part, however, this will not be possible and you should begin your preparation by deciding on the key message you wish to convey. Do not be tempted to try to cram all the available information into the time allocated as this may lead to a rushed presentation that fails to capture the attention of your audience.

Most contemporary presentations are prepared using PowerPoint or similar. For a presentation of less than 30 minutes, there should be a maximum of 15 slides (equivalent to one every two minutes). Key points should be displayed on each slide with no more than six per slide. Overcrowded slides mean the font sizes are too small and they are difficult to read. It is recommended that for ease of reading and accessibility font sizes should be 20 or above. In addition, when there is too much information on a slide you can lose the audience as they are focusing on trying to read what is on your slides rather than listen to what you are saying. If you have prepared well you should be sufficiently familiar with the material to be able to address each of the points with the aid of prompt cards or notes.

Other features that should be used with caution are vivid colour schemes, animated text and complex animations and transitions. While these can look impressive on a computer, when transferred to a projector they can be difficult to read and, if overused, can detract from the essential message. Help with preparing presentations may be available locally from the university or health service provider but assistance can also be found on the Internet.

Rehearsing is fundamental to ensuring that your final presentation is as polished as it can be. It also gives you the opportunity to ensure you are keeping to the allocated time. While a minute or two over time may not appear important, strict scheduling of sessions means that timing is important for the overall smooth running of the conference. Many conference organisers have timekeepers who may stop the presentation if you go over your allocated time and this can be frustrating for you and your audience.

Presenting to peers or colleagues is a good idea as you will be able to receive constructive feedback within a safe environment. It will also allow you to practise and seek comments on your delivery. It is very likely that you will be nervous when you are presenting and this can affect how you communicate verbally and non-verbally. With practice you can moderate both the clarity and the speed with which you speak, as well as rehearse how to assume a good posture and maintain eye-contact with your audience.

Many conference organisers require that the presentation is submitted before the conference begins. This allows presentations to be loaded onto the appropriate computer before the conference starts with the aim of facilitating the transition from one presentation to the next. However, you should ensure that you have a backup copy on a flash drive in the event of a technological problem. When you arrive at the conference you should visit the venue for your presentation and ensure you are familiar with the audiovisual equipment.

Preparing a Poster Presentation

An alternative means of presenting at a conference, seminar or workshop is through a poster presentation. Developing posters is a skill that many undergraduates develop during their educational programmes as they often form part of a module assessment. Thus, when presented with the opportunity to develop a poster for presentation, students may feel less fearful. Moreover, poster presentations at conferences are often located together in a given area where conference attendees can examine them at their leisure. This facilitates a mode of communication that is less formal and more relaxed.

The same criteria apply when submitting an abstract for a poster presentation as for an oral presentation. The selection panel will review the submission and inform you when it is accepted. The time needed to prepare a poster should not be underestimated and it is important to begin preparations once you have received the acceptance notification. Since you will not be able to include all the information from your review on the poster you will have to decide on the key message. Following this, the poster will have to be designed and possibly edited on more than one occasion before it is finally produced.

Seeking assistance with designing and producing a poster is recommended. Some universities and health service providers may be able to help with the design, following which you may be able to send it to a printer for a relatively small cost. The alternative is to design and produce the poster with the assistance of a professional graphic designer, although this can make the process expensive.

The conference organisers will have specified the size of the poster and it is important that you adhere to this so that it will fit the poster display units. General principles regarding the use of colour, typefaces and text are similar to those for an oral presentation using PowerPoint. Posters that are too busy, with strong colours, too much text and too many photographs or images can be difficult to read and detract from the overall message. Background and foreground colours should be chosen with care so that the text stands out clearly. Limiting the colours to two or three that complement each other is recommended. Typefaces should be limited to one or two and used consistently. Text should be presented concisely but preferably in blocks that can be read easily.

Despite the need to exercise caution about colour, typeface, text and content, your poster should still be sufficiently visually appealing to attract attention. Having a clearly visible title is important as conference attendees are likely to be viewing posters during breaks in conference proceedings. Therefore, they will have limited time and you need to grab their attention. Used judiciously, graphics, figures and photographs will add to the visual impact of the poster.

Whatever the setting in which you are presenting your poster, it is expected that you are available to answer any questions viewers may have. You should, therefore, be present at the poster at times when you know there are people likely to be viewing it. An unattended poster will receive less attention and removes the opportunity for you to showcase your work.

Summary

This chapter has provided a brief outline of some of the avenues you might pursue to disseminate or share the findings of a literature review that forms part of a dissertation or which has been submitted as an academic assignment. For the dissemination of systematic reviews, the reader is referred to CRD (2009), Bettany-Saltikov (2012) and Gough et al. (2012). These include submitting to a journal for publication or presenting a paper or poster at a conference, seminar or workshop.

🔑 **Key Points** 🔑

- A literature review may produce findings that are of interest to your discipline.
- Literature reviews that form part of a dissertation or have been written for an academic assignment have the potential to be published.
- Disseminating the findings of a literature review through publication in a journal or an oral presentation or poster at a conference, seminar or workshop has the potential to raise awareness, provoke discussion and identify implications for future practice, education and research in the area.

Glossary

Binary (dichotomous) data: Data in which there are only two categories – e.g. alive/dead, sick/well.

Citation: This is acknowledgement of another author's ideas or work by referring to or citing them as the source.

Concept: An abstract idea about a particular phenomenon.

Concept analysis: A method by which concepts that are of interest to any discipline are examined in order to clarify their characteristics, thereby achieving a better understanding of the meaning of that concept.

Conceptual framework: Concepts of similar meaning that provide a means for understanding a particular phenomenon and may be used to guide the analysis phase of a study.

Confidence interval: Used to express the degree of uncertainty associated with each result in a study.

Continuous data: Data that can have an infinite number of possible values – e.g. weight, area, volume.

Critical analysis: An appraisal of the quality of a research report. It differs from a critique in that only the significant strengths/limitations of the study are presented.

Critical appraisal: The critical analysis of a body of knowledge.

Critique: A critical examination of all aspects of a research report that identifies both the strengths and the limitations of that study.

Data: Information gleaned from a study.

Descriptive synthesis: The collation and presentation of information about each study included in a review. This is often presented as a tabular summary of key aspects. A descriptive synthesis of literature other than primary studies can also be collated and presented.

Dissemination: Most dictionary definitions refer to dissemination as 'scattering', 'spreading' or 'dispersing'. In the context of healthcare research and knowledge it is a planned process associated usually with informing others about the results of research studies. However, dissemination is not confined to the findings of research studies.

Effect measure: The observed relationship between an intervention and an outcome.

Ethnography: A qualitative research approach that has its origins in anthropology and studies group culture as a means of understanding behaviour.

Evidence-based medicine/evidence-based practice: Integrating the best available research evidence with clinical expertise and the individual patient's values and preferences in order to make decisions about that patient's care.

Fixed-effect model: A means of 'weighting' the contribution of a study to the overall summary estimate in a meta-analysis. Fixed-effect assumes one effect size with the result that studies that are larger and contain more information are given greater weighting than smaller studies.

Forest plot: A graphic display of the information from individual studies in a meta-analysis. It illustrates the amount of variation between studies and the overall result. It also displays the 'confidence interval' (see above) of each result.

Grounded theory: A qualitative research approach that attempts to generate a theory based on the data gathered from participants in a study.

Hierarchies of evidence: Some evidence is valued more highly than other evidence, based primarily on the type of research used to generate it. Randomised controlled trials (RCTs) are considered the 'gold standard', with qualitative studies rated as the least rigorous and reliable. This hierarchy is now seen as controversial.

Integrative literature review: Summarises and draws conclusions on past research on a given topic. Research is interpreted in its broadest sense and literature that is sourced can include primary research, and theoretical and conceptual literature.

Literature review: A critical evaluation of a subject. Used for research purposes, policy and practice development and for critical analysis of theoretical and conceptual frameworks.

Literature search: Searching for and identifying literature appropriate for addressing the research question.

Mean difference (weighted mean difference): The mean difference or 'difference in means' measures the absolute difference between the means in two groups. The difference represents the amount by which an intervention changes the outcome on average when compared with the control group.

Meta-analysis: A process of statistical analysis of numerical data where the findings of individual studies are pooled and re-analysed as one, bigger data set. The research designs and methods of the included studies must be reasonably homogeneous (similar) with the gold standard being RCTs. The outcome of such an exercise is to increase the power and the accuracy of the effect of an intervention.

Meta-ethnography: A synthesis of first- and second-order concepts to construct a new interpretation or theory about the phenomenon under study. First-order concepts are those identified by the participants in an individual study. Second-order concepts are the original researcher's interpretation of the first-order concepts. The main purpose of a meta-ethnography is to create a new or third-order interpretation.

Meta-study: An approach to the synthesis of qualitative research studies that has three analytic phases: meta-data analysis, meta-method and meta-theory. These three analytic strategies must be undertaken before meta-synthesis can occur. The aim is to generate new and more complete understandings of the phenomenon under study.

Meta-synthesis: A process whereby the findings from individual qualitative research studies are deconstructed (broken down), examined and reconstructed into a new interpretation.

Narrative/traditional/descriptive literature review: A literature review conducted to identify, analyse, assess and interpret a body of knowledge on a topic. The results of the review are presented narratively, usually in the form of themes.

Narrative synthesis: Similar to a thematic analysis in that it uses narrative to synthesise evidence. However, it differs in that it attempts to generate new knowledge or insights. The narrative involves an analysis of the relationships within and between studies and assesses the strength of the evidence.

Naturalistic: Associated with qualitative research, upholding the notion of multiple subjective realities that are constructed by individuals and are context bound.

Odds ratio: Assesses how likely it is that someone who is exposed to the factor under study will develop an outcome compared to someone who is not exposed. An odds ratio of 1 indicates no difference between the groups being compared.

Paraphrasing: Presenting another author's work or ideas in your own words. The original author must be acknowledged as the source.

Phenomenology: A philosophical movement that has had significant influence in the conduct of qualitative research. Phenomenology is concerned with the study of the lived experience.

Plagiarism: Taking another author's work and claiming it as your own. It most frequently occurs when writers fail to acknowledge another author's work that they have quoted or paraphrased.

Positivism: Is a paradigm (way of looking at the world) that is associated with the traditional method of scientific enquiry and quantitative research methods. Features of positivism include beliefs that an objective reality exists and can be measured. Positivism has largely been replaced with post-positivism, which is a more moderate extension of its philosophy.

Probability sampling: A quantitative sampling method in which all members of the population have an equal chance (greater than zero) of being selected. Random sampling methods are examples.

Purpose/aim: A clear statement that broadly identifies, both to the reader and the researcher, what is to be achieved. It is usually identified early in the work and acts as a signpost for the reader.

Qualitative meta-summary: A process of aggregating qualitative research findings through a quantitative process for the purpose of determining the frequency of each finding in and across studies.

Qualitative research: Research involving the subjective experiences and perceptions of participants. Data are not analysed statistically.

Quantitative research: Research that involves quantifying and measuring data statistically.

Quotation: Taking a segment of another author's work and presenting it word for word as it originally appeared. The quotation is presented in inverted commas or is indented in the text, and the original author is acknowledged by the reviewer.

Random-effect model: Another means of 'weighting' the contribution of a study to the overall summary statistic in a meta-analysis. Random-effect assumes that factors in the study such as the population in the study, implementation or measurement of the intervention result in variation in effect sizes across studies. This results in greater balance between larger and smaller studies.

Randomised controlled trial (RCT): An experiment that is designed to test the effectiveness of an intervention. In an RCT participants are randomly allocated to one of two groups. One group receives the intervention and the other does not. The results are compared between the two groups.

Realist literature review: Developed originally for complex social interventions to examine how context influences the relationship between an intervention and its outcome. Sometimes represented as context–mechanism–outcome (C–M–O), it focuses on discovering what works, how it works, for whom it works, the extent to which it works and under what conditions. To date, much of the focus of realist reviews is in the areas of health policy and practice.

References: A list of all the authors and their works referred to or quoted within a review, study or any written work.

Relative risk: Compares risk levels. In a study with two groups (one control and one intervention) the relative risk is the proportion of people in *both* groups who would experience the event. For example, the risk of developing lung cancer is much higher among smokers than non-smokers. Relative risk calculates this proportion. A relative risk of 1 indicates no difference between the groups being compared.

Research problem: An issue or question that needs further evidence to help resolve it. The problem can relate to practice or other issues, such as patients' knowledge or behaviour. In some situations the research problem may be identified by reviewing some of the literature associated with the research topic and identifying where there are gaps. Alternatively, a clinical or practice problem can sometimes help to identify a research topic.

Research question: A brief statement formulated as a question. There can be more than one presented in a study. It usually has a narrow focus and is frequently presented after the literature review. In a systematic review, however, a focused research question is needed to perform the review as, in essence, this type of review is a research study in its own right.

Research topic/phenomenon of interest: A broad area of interest, also called a concept, which forms the basis for a research study or literature review. In qualitative research it is sometimes identified as the phenomenon of interest.

Scoping literature review: A non-protocol driven literature review scopes the literature for a number of reasons that can include: mapping research activity in a given area; determining the feasibility of undertaking a full systematic review; summarising and disseminating research to interested groups; identifying gaps in the research; developing methodological/theoretical ideas for future research; justifying future research; and clarifying conceptual understanding. It differs from other types of review in that it does not formally appraise the quality of the research or make recommendations.

Standard deviation: A statistical measure of the dispersion or spread of data from the mean (average). Most data in a sample is what is known as 'normally distributed', which means that the results are close or reasonably close to the average. Standard deviation measures how tightly the results are spread around the average. The standard deviation is useful for determining how diverse the results are for a given study.

Standardised mean difference: Used as a summary statistic when a number of studies have measured the same outcome but does so in different ways. Because different measures are used, the findings have to be standardised before they can be pooled. This is done by examining the size of the effect of the intervention in each study against the variability. Variability is referred to as the 'standard deviation' (see above).

Systematic review: A process that uses an explicit and transparent methodology to re-analyse and synthesise evidence from previously conducted research studies on a given topic. Systematic reviews are generally classed as 'research on research' or secondary research because they do not collect new data but use the findings from previous research.

Thematic analysis: A process whereby findings are summarised and synthesised and presented as a narrative using identified themes. The focus is primarily on providing a summary rather than new insight. Findings are generally preserved in their original form.

Theme: A unit of meaning that occurs regularly in data.

Theoretical sampling: A form of purposive sampling used in grounded theory, with participants selected on the basis of emerging study data.

Variable: Something that can change between different situations or different individuals – e.g. body temperature.

Theory: Assumptions and knowledge pertaining to a topic.

Theoretical framework: Underlying theory pertaining to a specific topic that serves to contextualise a literature review.

References

Akerjordet, K. and Severinsson, E. (2007) 'Emotional intelligence: a review of the literature with specific focus on empirical and epistemological perspectives', *Journal of Clinical Nursing*, 16 (8): 1405–16.

Anderson, S., Allen, P., Peckham, S. and Goodwin, N. (2008) 'Asking the right questions: scoping studies in the commissioning of research on the organisation and delivery of health services', *Health Research Policy and Systems*, 6 (7), available at: www.health-policy-systems.com/content/6/1/7 (accessed: 20 December 2011).

Arai, L., Britten, N., Popay, J., Roberts, H., Petticrew, M., Rodgers, M. and Sowden, A. (2009) 'Testing methodological developments in the conduct of narrative synthesis: a demonstration review of research on the implementation of smoke alarm interventions', *Evidence and Policy*, 3 (3): 361–83.

Arksey, H. and O'Malley, L. (2005) 'Scoping studies: towards a methodological framework, *International Journal of Social Research Methodology*, 8 (1): 19–32.

Atkins, S., Lewin, S., Smith, H., Engel, M., Fretheim, A. and Volmink, J. (2008) 'Conducting a meta-ethnography of qualitative literature: lessons learnt, *BMC Medical Research Methodology*, 8 (21), available at: http://biomedcentral.com/1471-2288/8/21.

Aveyard, H. (2010) *Doing a Literature Review in Health and Social Care: A Practical Guide.* 2nd edn. Maidenhead: Open University Press.

Barnett-Page, E. and Thomas, J. (2009) 'Methods for the synthesis of qualitative research: a critical review', *BMC Medical Research Methodology*, 9 (59), available at: www.biomedcentral.com/1471-2288/9/59.

Beauchamp, T.L. and Childress J.F. (2009) *Principles of Biomedical Ethics.* 6th edn. Oxford: Oxford University Press.

Beck, C.T. (2002) 'Postpartum depression: a metasynthesis', *Qualitative Health Research*, 12: 453–71.

Beecroft, C., Rees, A. and Booth, A. (2006) 'Finding the evidence', in K. Gerrish and A. Lacey (eds) *The Research Process in Nursing.* 5th edn. Oxford: Blackwell Publishing Ltd.

Belgrave, L., Zablotsky, D. and Guadagno, M.A. (2002) 'How do we talk to each other? Writing qualitative research for quantitative readers', *Qualitative Health Research*, 12: 1427–39.

Benton,D. and Cormack, D. (1996) 'Reviewing and evaluating the literature', in D. Cormack, (ed.) *The Research Process in Nursing.* 3rd edition. Oxford: Blackwell Science Ltd.

Berkhof, M., van Rijssen, H.J., Schellart, A.J.M., Anema, J.R. and van der Beek, A.J. (2011) 'Effective training strategies for teaching communication skills to physicians: an overview of systematic reviews', *Patient Education and Counseling*, 84: 152–62.

Bettany-Saltikov, J. (2012) *How to Do a Systematic Literature Review in Nursing. A Step-by-Step Guide.* Maidenhead: Open University Press.

Bissonnette, J. (2008) 'Adherence: a concept analysis', *Journal of Advanced Nursing*, 63 (6): 634–43.

Boehm, K., Borrelli, F., Ernst, E., Habacher, G., Hung, S.K., Milazzo, S. and Horneber, M. (2009) 'Green tea (Camellia sinensis) for the prevention of cancer', *Cochrane Database of Systematic Reviews 2009*, 3: Art. no.: CD005004. DOI: 10.1002/14651858.CD005004. pub2, available at: www.cochrane.org/cochrane-reviews (accessed: 23 November 2011).

Bondas, T., Hall, E.O.C. (2007) 'A decade of metasynthesis research in health sciences: a meta-method study', *International Journal of Qualitative Studies on Health and Well-being*, 2: 101–13.

Booth, A., Rees, A. and Beecroft, C. (2010) 'Systematic reviews and evidence synthesis', in K. Gerrish and A. Lacey (eds) *The Research Process in Nursing.* 6th edn. Oxford: Wiley-Blackwell. pp. 284–302.

Broome, M.E. (2000) 'Integrative literature reviews for the development of concepts', in B.L. Rodgers and K.A. Knafl (eds) *Concept Development in Nursing: Foundations, Techniques and Applications.* 2nd edn. Philadelphia: Saunders. pp. 231–50.

Brouwers, M., Kho, M.E., Browman, G.P., Burgers, J.S., Cluzeau, F., Feder, G., Fervers, B., Graham, ID., Grimshaw, J., Hanna, S., Littlejohns, P., Makarski, J. and Zitzelsberger, L. for the AGREE Next Steps Consortium (2010) 'AGREE II: advancing guideline development, reporting and evaluation in healthcare', *Canadian Medical Association Journal*, 182: E839-842. DOI: 10.1503/090449.

Brunton, G., Wiggins, M. and Oakley, A. (2011) *Becoming a Mother: a Research Synthesis of Women's Views on the Experience of First-time Motherhood.* London: EPPI Centre, Social Science Research Unit, Institute of Education, University of London.

Burns, N. and Grove, S.K. (2007) *Understanding Nursing Research: Building an Evidence-Based Practice.* 4th edn. St Louis, MO: Saunders Elsevier.

Campbell, R., Pound, P., Morgan, M., Daker-White, G., Britten, N., Pill, R., Yardley, L., Pope, C. and Donovan, J. (2011) 'Evaluating meta-ethnography: systematic analysis and synthesis of qualitative research', *Health Technology Assessment*, 15 (43): ISSN 1366–5278.

Carnwell, R. and Daly, W. (2001) 'Strategies for the construction of a critical review of the literature', *Nurse Education in Practice*, 1: 57–63.

Catling-Paull, C., Johnston, R., Ryan, C., Foureur, M.J. and Homer, C.S.E. (2011) 'Clinical interventions that increase the uptake and success of vaginal birth after caesarean section: a systematic review', *Journal of Advanced Nursing*, 67 (8): 1646–61.

Centre for Reviews and Dissemination (CRD) (2009) *Systematic Reviews: CRD's Guidance for Undertaking Reviews in Health Care.* York: CRD, University of York.

Clarke, M. (2006) 'Systematic review and meta-analysis of quantitative research: overview of methods' (part 1, chapter 1), in: C. Webb and B. Roe (eds) *Reviewing Research Evidence for Nursing Practice: Systematic Reviews.* Oxford: Blackwell Publishing. pp. 3–8.

Cohen, G. (1990) 'Memory', in: I. Roth (ed.) *The Open University's Introduction to Psychology.* Volume 2. Milton Keynes: Lawrence Erlbaum.

Conkin Dale, J. (2005) 'Critiquing research for use in practice', *Journal of Pediatric Health Care*, 19: 183–6.

Coughlan, M., Cronin, P. and Ryan, F. (2007) 'Step-by-step guide to critiquing research. Part 1: quantitative research', *British Journal of Nursing*, 16 (11): 658–63.

Critical Appraisal Skills Programme (CASP) (2010), available at www.caspinternational. org/?o1020 (accessed: 23 March 2012).

Cronin, P. and Rawlings-Anderson, K. (2004) *Knowledge for Contemporary Nursing Practice.* Edinburgh: Mosby.

Cronin, P., Ryan, F. and Coughlan, M. (2008) 'Undertaking a literature review: a step-by-step approach', *British Journal of Nursing*, 17 (1): 38–43.

Cronin, P., Ryan, F. and Coughlan, M. (2010) 'Concept analysis in healthcare research', *International Journal of Therapy and Rehabilitation*, 17 (2): 62–8.

Davids, J.R., Weigl, D.M., Edmonds, J.P. and Blackhurst, D.W. (2010) 'Reference accuracy in peer-reviewed pediatric orthopaedic literature', *Journal of Bone and Joint Surgery (American Volume)*, 92 (5): 1155–1161.

Davis, K., Drey, N. and Gould, D. (2009) 'What are scoping studies? A review of the nursing literature', *International Journal of Nursing Studies*, 46: 1386–1400.

Downe, S. (2008) 'Metasynthesis: a guide to knitting smoke', *Evidence Based Midwifery*, 6 (1): 4–8.

Ely, C. and Scott, I. (2007) *Essential Study Skills for Nursing.* Edinburgh: Mosby.

Engberg, S. (2008) 'Systematic reviews and meta-analysis', *Journal of Wound Ostomy Continence Nursing*, 35 (3): 258–65.

Engwall, M. and Sorensen Duppils, G. (2009) 'Music as a nursing intervention for postoperative pain: a systematic review', *Journal of PeriAnesthesia Nursing*, 24 (6): 370–83.

Evans, D. (2002) 'Database searches for qualitative research', *Journal of the Medical Library Association*, 90 (3): 290–3.

Evans, D. (2003) 'Hierarchy of evidence: a framework for ranking evidence evaluating healthcare interventions', *Journal of Clinical Nursing*, 12: 77–84.

Evidence for Policy and Practice Information and Co-ordinating Centre (EPPI Centre) (2010) *EPPI-Centre Methods for Conducting Systematic Reviews*. London: EPPI-Centre, Social Science Research Unit, Institute of Education, University of London, available at: http://eppi.ioe.ac.uk/cms/Default.aspx?tabid=1915 (accessed: 20 October 2011).

Fellowes, D., Wilkinson, S. and Moore, P. (2004) 'Communication skills training for health care professionals working with cancer patients, their families and/or carers', *Cochrane Database Systematic Reviews 2004*: CD003751.

Finfgeld-Connett, D. (2010) 'Generalizability and transferability of meta-synthesis research findings', *Journal of Advanced Nursing*, 66 (2): 246–54.

Finfgeld, D.L. (2003) 'Metasynthesis: state of the art – so far', *Qualitative Health Research*, 13 (7): 893–904.

Finfgeld-Connett, D.L. (2008) 'Meta-synthesis of caring in nursing', *Journal of Clinical Nursing*, 17: 196–204.

Finlayson, K. and Dixon, A. (2008) 'Qualitative meta-synthesis: a guide for the novice', *Nurse Researcher*, 15 (2): 59–71.

Flemming, K. (2007) 'Synthesis of qualitative research and evidence-based nursing', *British Journal of Nursing*, 16 (10): 616–20.

Fored, C., Ejerbladm E., Lindblad, P., Fryzek, J., Dickman, P., Signorello, L., Lipworth, L., Elinder, C., Blot, W., McLaughlin, J., Zack, M. and Nyren, O. (2001) 'Acetaminophen, aspirin, and chronic renal failure', *New England Journal of Medicine*, 345: 1801–8.

Gerrish, K. and Lacey, A. (2010) 'Disseminating research findings', in K. Gerrish and A. Lacey (eds) *The Research Process in Nursing*. 6th edn. Wiley-Blackwell: Oxford. pp. 475–87.

Gough, D., Oliver, S. and Thomas, J. (2012) *An Introduction to Systematic Reviews*. London: Sage.

Gould, D. (2008) 'Undertaking a literature review project: guidance for nursing students', *Nursing Standard*, 22 (50): 48–54.

Grant, M., Cavanagh, A. and Yorke, J. (2012) 'The impact of caring for those with chronic obstructive pulmonary disease (COPD) on carers' psychological well-being: a narrative review', *International Journal of Nursing Studies*. DOI: 10.1016/j.ijnurstu.2012.02.010.

Greenhalgh, T. and Peacock, R. (2005) 'Effectiveness and efficiency of search methods in systematic reviews of complex evidence: audit of primary sources', *British Medical Journal*, 331 (7524): 1064–5.

Greenhalgh, T., Kristjansson, E. and Robinson, V. (2007) 'Realist review to understand the efficacy of school feeding programmes', *British Medical Journal*, 335: 858–61.

Greenhalgh, T., Wong G., Westhorp, G. and Pawson, R. (2011) 'Protocol – realist and meta-narrative evidence synthesis: evolving standards (RAMESES)', *BioMed Central Medical Research Methodology*, 11: 115, available at: www.biomedcentral.com/1471-2288/11/115 (accessed: 28 December 2011).

Guyatt, G., Cook, D. and Haynes, B. (2004) 'Evidence based medicine has come a long way', *British Medical Journal*, 329: 390–1.

Hamer, S. and Collinson G. (2005) *Achieving Evidence-based Practice. A Handbook for Practitioners*. 2nd edn. Edinburgh: Ballière Tindall.

Hardy, S. and Ramjeet, J. (2005) 'Reflections on how to write and organise a research thesis', *Nurse Researcher*, 13 (2): 27–39.

Hart, C. (2010) *Doing a Literature Review. Releasing the Social Science Research Imagination*. London: Sage.

Hawker, S., Payne, S., Kerr, C., Hardley, M. and Powell, J. (2002) 'Appraising the evidence: reviewing disparate data systematically', *Qualitative Health Research*, 12 (9): 1289–99.

Hek, G. and Langton, H. (2000) 'Systematically searching and reviewing literature', *Nurse Researcher*, 7 (3): 40–57.

Higgins, J.P.T. and Green, S. (eds) (2008) *Cochrane Handbook for Systematic Reviews of Interventions*. Chichester: Wiley-Blackwell.

Jones, J. (2005) 'Evaluation of pressure ulcer prevention devices: a critical review of the literature', *Journal of Wound Care*, 14 (9): 422–5.

Jones, K. (2005) 'Diversities in approach to end-of-life care: a view from Britain of the qualitative literature', *Journal of Research in Nursing*, 10: 431–53.

Koch, T. (2006) 'Establishing rigour in qualitative research: the decision trail', *Journal of Advanced Nursing*, 53 (1): 91–103.

Kristjansson, B., Petticrew, M. and MacDonald, B. (2007) 'School feeding for improving the physical and psychosocial health of disadvantaged students', *Cochrane Database of Systematic Reviews 2007*, 1: Art. no.: CD004676. DOI: 10.1002/14651858.CD004676. pub2, available at: www.cochrane.org/cochrane-reviews (accessed: 29 December 2011).

Kübler-Ross, E. (1969) *On Death and Dying*. New York: Macmillan.

Lahlafi, A. (2007) 'Conducting a literature review: how to carry out bibliographical database searches', *British Journal of Cardiac Nursing*, 2 (12): 566–9.

Lane, C. and Rollnick, S. (2007) 'The use of simulated patients and role-play in communication skills training: a review of the literature to August 2005', *Patient Education and Counseling*, 67: 13–20.

Larun, L. and Malterud, K. (2007) 'Identity and coping experiences in Chronic Fatigue Syndrome: a synthesis of qualitative studies', *Patient Education and Counseling*, 69: 20–8.

Law, J. and Plunkett, C. (2009) 'The interaction between behaviour and speech and language difficulties: does intervention for one affect outcomes in the other? Technical report', in *Research Evidence in Education Library*. London: EPPI-Centre, Social Science Research Unit, Institute of Education, University of London, available at: http://eppi.ioe.ac.uk/cms/ (accessed: 23 November 2011).

Lee, P. (2006) 'Understanding and critiquing quantitative research papers', *Nursing Times*, 102 (28): 28–30.

Lindahl, B. and Lindblad, B.M. (2011) 'Family members' experiences of everyday life when a child is dependent on a ventilator: a metasynthesis study', *Journal of Family Nursing*, 17: 241–69.

Machi, L. and McEvoy, B. (2009) *The Literature Review: Six Steps to Success*. Thousand Oaks, CA: Sage.

Madden, S.G., Loeb, S.J. and Smith, C.A. (2008) 'An integrative literature review of lifestyle interventions for the prevention of type II diabetes mellitus', *Journal of Clinical Nursing*, 17: 2243–56.

Marshall, J., Goldbart, J., Pickstone, C. and Roulstone, S. (2011) 'Application of systematic reviews in speech-and-language therapy', *International Journal of Language and Communication Disorders*, 46 (3): 261–72.

Maxwell, J.A. (2006) 'Literature reviews of, and for, educational research: a commentary on Boote and Beile's "Scholars Before Researchers"', *Educational Researcher*, 35 (9): 28–31.

Mays, N., Pope, C. and Popay, J. (2005) 'Systematically reviewing qualitative and quantitative evidence to inform management and policy-making in the health field', *Journal of Health Services Research and Policy*, 10 (Suppl. 1): 6–20.

McCabe, M. (2009) 'Fatigue in children with long-term conditions: an evolutionary concept analysis', *Journal of Advanced Nursing*, 65 (8): 1735–45.

Moher, D., Liberati, A., Tetzlaff, J., Altman, D.G. and The PRISMA Group (2009) 'Preferred reporting items for systematic reviews and meta-analyses: the PRISMA Statement', *PLoS Med* 6 (6), available at: http://medicine.plosjournals.org/ (accessed: 10 April 2012).

Montori, V.M., Wilczynski, N.L., Morgan, D. and Haynes, R.B. (2005) 'Optimal search strategies for retrieving systematic reviews from Medline: analytical survey', *British Medical Journal*, 330 (7482): 68–71.

Morse, J.M. (2009) 'Mixing qualitative methods', *Qualitative Health Research*, 19 (11): 1523–4.

Muir Gray, J.A. (2001) *Evidence-based Health Care*. Edinburgh: Churchill Livingstone.

Nepal, V.P. (2010) 'On mixing qualitative methods', *Qualitative Health Research*, 20 (2): 281.

Noblit, G.W. and Hare, R.D. (1988) *Meta-ethnography: Synthesising Qualitative Studies*. London: Sage.

Oermann, M.H., Galvin, E.A., Floyd, J.A. and Roop, J.C. (2006) 'Presenting research to clinicians: strategies for writing about research findings, *Nurse Researcher*, 13 (4): 66–74.

O'Malley, L. and Croucher, K. (2005) 'Housing and dementia care – a scoping review of the literature', *Health and Social Care in the Community*, 13 (6): 570–7.

Parahoo, K. (2006) *Nursing Research, Principles, Process and Issues*. 2nd edn. London: Palgrave.

Paterson, B., Canam, C., Joachim, G. and Thorne, S. (2003) 'Embedded assumptions in qualitative studies of fatigue', *Western Journal of Nursing Research*, 25 (2): 119–133.

Paterson, B., Dubouloz, C.J., Chevrier, J., Ashe, B., King, J. and Moldoveanu, M. (2009) 'Conducting qualitative metasynthesis research: insights from a metasynthesis project', *International Journal of Qualitative Methods*, 8 (3): 22–33.

Paterson, B., Thorne, S., Canam, C. and Jillings, C. (2001) *Meta-Study of Qualitative Health Research. A Practical Guide to Meta-Analysis and Meta-Synthesis*. Thousand Oaks, CA: Sage.

Patrick, L.J. and Munroe, S. (2004) 'The literature review: demystifying the literature search', *The Diabetes Educator*, 30: 30–38.

Pawson, R., Greenhalgh, T., Harvey, G. and Walshe, K. (2005) 'Realist review – a new method of systematic review designed for complex policy interventions', *Journal of Health Services Research and* Policy, 10 (Suppl. 1): 21–34.

Pickles, D., King, L. and Belan, I. (2009) 'Attitudes of nursing students towards caring for people with HIV/AIDS: thematic literature review', *Journal of Advanced Nursing*, 65 (11): 2262–73.

Pinto, R.A., Holanda, M.A., Medeiros, M.M.C., Mota, R.M.S. and Pereira, E.D.B. (2007) 'Assessment of the burden of caregiving for patients with chronic obstructive pulmonary disease', *Respiratory Medicine*, 101 (11): 2402–8.

Piquero, A., Farrington, D., Welsh, B., Tremblay, R. and Jennings, W. (2008) 'Effects of early family/parent training programs on antisocial behavior and delinquency', *Campbell Collaboration*, available at: www.campbellcollaboration.org/library.php (accessed: 23 November 2011).

Polit, D.F. and Beck, C.T. (2006) *Essentials of Nursing Research. Methods, Appraisal and Utilisation*. 6th edn. Philadelphia: Lippincott Williams & Wilkins.

Polit, D.F. and Beck, C.T. (2012) *Nursing Research: Generating and Assessing Evidence for Nursing Practice*. 9th edn. Philadelphia: Wolters Kluwer Health/Lippincott Williams & Wilkins.

Popay, J., Roberts, H., Sowden, A., Petticrew, M., Arai, L. and Rodgers, M. (2006) *Guidance on the Conduct of Narrative Synthesis in Systematic Reviews. Final report*. Swindon: ESRC Methods Programme.

Price, B. (2009) 'Guidance on conducting a literature search and reviewing mixed literature', *Nursing Standard*, 23 (24): 43–9.

Price, B. (2010) 'Disseminating best practice through publication in journals', *Nursing Standard*, 24 (26): 35–41.

Price, S.L. (2009) 'Becoming a nurse: a meta-study of early professional socialization and career choice in nursing', *Journal of Advanced Nursing*, 65 (1): 11–19.

Raijmakers, N.J., van Zuylen, L., Costantini, M., Caraceni, A., Clark, J., Lundquist, G., Voltz, R., Ellershaw, J.E., van der Heide, A. and on behalf of OPCARE9 (2011) 'Artificial nutrition and hydration in the last week of life in cancer patients: a systematic literature review of practices and effects', *Annals of Oncology*, 22 (7): 1478–86.

Rebar, C.R., Gersch, C.J., MacNee, C.L. and McCabe, S. (2011) *Understanding Nursing Research*. 3rd edn. Philadelphia: Wolters Kluwer Health/Lippincott Williams & Wilkins.

Rees, R., Oliver, K., Woodman, J. and Thomas, J. (2009) 'Children's views about obesity, body size, shape and weight: a systematic review', in *Research Evidence in Education Library*. London: EPPI-Centre, Social Science Research Unit, Institute of Education, University of London, available at: http://eppi.ioe.ac.uk/cms (accessed: 23 November 2011).

Ridley, D. (2008) *The Literature Review: A Step-by-Step Guide for Students*. Los Angeles: Sage.

Ring, N., Ritchie, K., Mandava, L. and Jepson, R. (2010) 'A guide to synthesising qualitative research for researchers undertaking health technology assessments and systematic reviews', *NHS Quality Improvement Scotland*, available at: www.nhshealthquality.org/nhsqis/8837.html (accessed 3 May 2012).

Rodgers, B.L. and Knafl, K.A. (2000) *Concept Development in Nursing*. 2nd edn. Philadelphia: Saunders.

Rodgers, M., Sowden, A., Petticrew, M., Arai, L., Roberts, H., Britten, N. and Popay, J. (2009) 'Testing methodological guidance on the conduct of narrative synthesis in systematic reviews', *Evaluation*, 15 (1): 47–71.

Ryan, F., Coughlan, M. and Cronin, P. (2007) 'Step-by-step guide to critiquing research. Part 2: qualitative research', *British Journal of Nursing*, 16 (12): 738–44.

Ryan-Wenger, N. (1992) 'Guidelines for critique of a research report', *Heart and Lung*, 21 (4): 394–401.

Sackett, D.L., Rosenberg, W.M.C., Muir Gray, J.A., Haynes, R.B. and Scott Richardson, W. (1996) 'Evidence based medicine: what it is and what it isn't', *British Medical Journal*, 312 (7023): 71.

Sandelowski, M. and Barroso, J. (2003a) 'Classifying the findings in qualitative studies', *Qualitative Health Research*, 13: 905–23.

Sandelowski, M. and Barroso, J. (2003b) 'Creating metasummaries of qualitative findings', *Nursing Research*, 52 (4): 226–33.

Sandelowski, M. and Barroso, J. (2007) *Handbook for Synthesizing Qualitative Research*. New York: Springer.

Sandelowski, M., Barroso, J. and Voils, C.I. (2007) 'Using qualitative metasummary to synthesize qualitative and quantitative descriptive findings', *Research in Nursing & Health*, 30: 99–111.

Seamark, D.A., Blake, S.D., Seamark, C.J. and Halpin, D.M. (2004) 'Living with severe chronic obstructive pulmonary disease (COPD): perceptions of patients and their carers. An interpretative phenomenological analysis', *Palliative Medicine*, 18 (7): 619–25.

Shea, B.J., Grimshaw, J.M., Wells, G.A., Boers, M., Andersson, N., Hamel, C., Porter, A.C., Tugwell, P., Moher, D. and Bouter, L.M. (2007) 'Development of AMSTAR: a measurement tool to assess the methodological quality of systematic reviews', *BioMed Central Medical Research Methodology*, 7 (10), available at: www.biomedcentral.com/1471-2288/7/10 (accessed: 23 November 2011).

Shepperd, S., McClaran, J., Phillips, C.O., Lannin, N.A., Clemson, L.M., McCluskey, A., Cameron, I.D. and Barras, S.L. (2010) 'Discharge planning from hospital to home', *Cochrane Database of Systematic Reviews 2010*, 1: Art. no.: CD000313. DOI: 10.1002/14651858.CD000313.pub3.

Shields, M. (2010) *Essay Writing. A Student's Guide*. London: Sage.

Singer, P., Martin, D. and Kelner, M. (1999) 'Quality end-of-life care: patients' perspectives', *Journal of the American Medical Association*, 281: 163–68.

Spilsbury, K., Hewitt, C. and Bowman, C. (2011) 'The relationship between nurse staffing and quality of care in nursing homes: a systematic review', *International Journal of Nursing Studies*, 48: 732–50.

Streubert Speziale, H.J. and Carpenter, D.R. (2007) *Qualitative Research in Nursing. Advancing the Humanistic Imperative.* 4th edn. Philadelphia: Lippincott Williams & Wilkins.

Stroup, D.F., Berlin, J.A., Morton, S.C., Olkin, I., Williamson, G.D., Rennie, D., Moher, D., Becker, B.J., Sipe, T.A. and Thacker, S.B. (2000) 'Meta-analysis of observational studies in epidemiology: a proposal for reporting. Meta-analysis of Observational Studies in Epidemiology (MOOSE) group', *JAMA*, 283 (15): 2008–12.

Tait, M. and Slater, J. (1999) 'Using computers in nursing research', *Nurse Researcher*, 7 (1): 17–29.

Thorne, S., Paterson, B., Acorn, S., Canam, C., Joachim, G. and Jillings, C. (2002) 'Chronic illness experience: insights from a metastudy', *Qualitative Research*, 12 (4): 437–52.

Timmins, F. and McCabe, C. (2005) 'How to conduct an effective literature review', *Nursing Standard*, 20 (11): 41–7.

Torraco, R.J. (2005) 'Writing integrative literature reviews: guidelines and examples', *Human Resource Development Review*, 4 (3): 356–67.

Truss, L. (2003) *Eats, Shoots & Leaves: the Zero Tolerance Approach to Punctuation.* London: Profile Books.

University of Queensland Library (2012) *Referencing Styles*, available at: www.library.uq.edu.au/infoskil/styles2.html (accessed: 16 July 2012).

Walker, J. (2010) 'Measuring plagiarism: researching what students do, not what they say they do', *Studies in Higher Education*, 35 (1): 41–59.

Walker, L. and Avant, K. (2011) *Strategies for Theory Construction in Nursing.* 5th edn. Norwalk, CT: Appleton & Lange.

Walsh, D. and Downe, S. (2005) 'Meta-synthesis method for qualitative research: a literature review', *Journal of Advanced Nursing*, 50 (2): 204–11.

Warren, M. (2009) 'Metastatic breast cancer recurrence: a literature review of themes and issues arising from diagnosis', *International Journal of Palliative Nursing*, 15 (5): 222–5.

Whiting, L.S. (2009) 'Systematic review protocols: an introduction', *Nurse Researcher*, 17 (1): 34–43.

Whittaker, A. and Williamson, G.R. (2011) *Succeeding in Research Project Plans and Literature Reviews for Nursing Students.* Exeter: Learning Matters.

Whittemore, R. (2005) 'Analysis of integration in nursing science and practice', *Journal of Nursing Scholarship*, 37 (3): 261–7.

Whittemore, R. and Knafl, K. (2005) 'The integrative review: updated methodology', *Journal of Advanced Nursing*, 52 (5): 546–53.

Williams, A. and Manias, E. (2008) 'A structured literature review of pain assessment and management of patients with kidney disease', *Journal of Clinical Nursing*, 17: 69–81.

Wright, J.M. and Musini, V.M. (2009) 'First-line drugs for hypertension', available at: www.cochrane.org/cochrane-reviews, *Cochrane Database of Systematic Reviews 2009*, 3: Art. no.: CD001841. DOI: 10.1002/14651858.CD001841.pub2 (accessed: 23 November 2011).

Zafron, M.L. (2012) 'Good intentions: providing students with skills to avoid accidental plagiarism', *Medical Reference Services Quarterly*, 31 (2): 225–9.

Index

This index is in word-by-word order. Page references in *italics* indicate figures and those in **bold** indicate tables.

abbreviations 117
abstracts 74, 112
acronyms 117
American Psychological Association (APA) referencing system 125–126
AMSTAR (assessment of multiple systematic reviews) 94, **95**
Appraisal of Guidelines for Research and Evaluation II (AGREE II) 88
Assessment of Multiple Systematic Reviews (AMSTAR) 8
authors 73
autonomy 77

believability
    See credibility (believability)
beneficence 77
bibliographical software packages 67–68
binary data (dichotomous data) 100

The Campbell Collaboration 12
catalogues 54
Centre for Reviews and Dissemination (CRD) 11, 20–21, 36, 43, 46
CINAHL (database) 57–59
Cochrane Centre in Oxford (now UK Cochrane Centre) 11
The Cochrane Collaboration 11, 12, 46
Cochrane Handbook for Systematic Reviews of Interventions (Higgins and Green) 35, 43
comparators 35
concept analysis 23–26, **24**
conceptual frameworks 75, 82
conclusions 84, 87, 115
conferences 132–135
confidentiality 77, 83
constant comparative analysis 104–105
credibility (believability)
    qualitative research and **79**, 80–84
    quantitative research and 72–74, **72**
critical analysis
    in literature reviews 88–89
    non-research literature and 88, **88**
    overview 69–71
    qualitative research and 79–84, **79–80**

critical analysis *cont.*
    quantitative research and 71–78, **72–73**
    systematic reviews and 85–87, **86**
Critical Appraisal Skills Programme (CASP) 8, 42, 66, 71, 86

data analysis
    concept analysis and 24
    critical analysis and 83
    vs. data synthesis 44
    integrative reviews and 17–18
    quantitative research and 78
data synthesis
    concept analysis and 24
    methods of 96–109, **96**, **97**
    overview 90–96, **91–96**
    realist reviews and 28
    systematic reviews and 43–45
    See also specific methods
databases
    literature search and 9–10, 53–54, **54**, 56–60, **58**
    systematic reviews and 85–86
definitions 76–77
descriptive reviews
    See narrative reviews
descriptive statistics 78
descriptive synthesis 91
dichotomous data (binary data) 100
dictionaries 55
discussions 78, 84

EBSCOhost 57
Economic and Social Research Council (ESRC) Methods Programme 98–99
effect measures 100–101
EndNote (bibliographical software) 67–68
EQUATOR network (Enhancing the Quality and Transparency of Health Research) 46
essays 4–5
ethical principles 77, 83
ethnography 81
evidence 12–14
evidence-based healthcare (EBH) 10
evidence-based medicine movement (EBM) 10

evidence-based practice (EBP) 10–12
Evidence for Policy and Practice Information and
    Co-ordinating Centre (EPPI-Centre) 11–12,
    42, 43, 46
experiential/practice literature 52
exploratory essays 4

fidelity 77
fixed-effect model 101
forest plot 102, *102*

generalisability 79
grammar 117
grey literature 55, 85
GreyNet (database) 55
grounded theory 81, 104

Harvard referencing system 125
holism 79

IMRAD (Introduction, Methods, Results,
    Discussion) 66
Index to Theses (database) 55
inferential statistics 78
integrative reviews 16–19
integrity (robustness)
    qualitative research and **79–80**, 80–84
    quantitative research and 72, **72–73**, 74–78
    systematic reviews and 85–87, **86**
Internet 53–54
interventions 35
introduction 112–113

jargon 117
journal articles 130–132
judgement essays 4
justice 77

keywords 57–58, 85

line of argument (LOA) synthesis 104–105
literature
    note taking and 67
    organization of 67
    reading and summary of 64–66
    selection of 62–64
    sources of 52–53
    types of 52
literature reviews
    critical analysis in 88–89
    definition of 1–2
    vs. essays 5
    purpose and importance of 2–4
    in qualitative research studies 2–3, 81–82
    in quantitative research studies 2–3, 75
    steps of 5–7
    types of 8–9, 13–14

literature search
    concept analysis and 24
    databases and 9–10, 53–54, **54**, 56–60, **58**
    integrative reviews and 17
    vs. literature reviews 2
    manual searches and 55–56
    narrative reviews and 15
    realist reviews and 27–28
    scoping reviews and 21
    systematic reviews and 38–40, 85–86
logical consistency 74

manual searches 55–56
mean difference (weighted mean difference) 101
MEDLINE (database) 54, 57–58
MeSH (Medical Subject Headings) 57
meta-analysis 44, 87, 100–102, *102*
Meta-analysis Of Observational Studies in
    Epidemiology (MOOSE) 46
meta-ethnography 45, 103–105, **105**
meta-study 103, 105–107, *106*
meta-synthesis
    methods of 103–107, **105**, *106*
    overview 45, 102–103
    qualitative systematic reviews and 87
    thematic analysis and 97–98, **97**
methodological relevance 42
methodology 76, 82
moral rules 77

narrative integration 87
narrative reviews 13, 14–16, 91
narrative synthesis 44–45, 98–99
National Institute for Health
    Research 11
non-maleficence 77, 83
note taking 67

odds ratio 100
operational definitions 76–77
outcomes 35–36

papers 132–134
paraphrasing 122, 124
PEO (population, exposure, outcomes) 34, 38,
    43, 92
phenomenology 81
philosophical literature 52
PICOS (population, interventions, comparators,
    outcomes and study design) 34–37, 38,
    43, 92
plagiarism 116, 123–124
policy literature 52
population 34–35
poster presentations 134–135
PQRS system (Preview, Question, Read,
    Summarise) 66

Preferred Reporting Items for Systematic Reviews and Meta-Analyses (PRISMA) 46, 92
privacy 77
process consent 83
Procite (bibliographical software) 67–68
PubMed (database) 57–58

qualitative meta-summary 103, 107–109
qualitative research
    critique of 79–84, **79–80**
    data synthesis and 45
    literature reviews and 2–3, 81–82
    vs. quantitative research 63, 115
    systematic reviews and 32–33, 36, 42, 87
quality assessment 41–43
quantitative research
    critique of 71–78, **72–73**
    data synthesis and 45
    literature reviews and 2–3, 75
    vs. qualitative research 63, 115
    systematic reviews and 36, 41–42, 87
quotations 121–122

random-effect model 101
randomised controlled trials (RCTs) 12–13, 30, 36, 44
realist reviews (realist synthesis) 27–29
reciprocal translational analysis (RTA) 104–105
recommendations 115–116
Reference Manager (bibliographical software) 67–68
references
    citations conventions and 124–127
    overview 116, 119–121
    paraphrasing and 122, 124
    qualitative research and 84
    quantitative research and 78
    quotations and 121–122
    systematic reviews and 87
reflective essays 4–5
refutational synthesis 104–105
relative risk 100
reliability 76
research designs 76, 82
research literature 52, 63
research methods 76, 82
research problems 74, 85
research questions
    critical analysis and 75–76
    overview 3
    selection of literature and 63–64
    systematic reviews and 34–37, 85
Review Manager (RevMan) 102
rigour 84

sampling 77, 82–83
scoping reviews 19–22, 33
search engines 53–54
Service Delivery and Organisation Research and Development programme (SDO Programme) 19–20
snowball technique 55
Social Science Research Institute, London 11
spelling 117
SQ3R Reading Technique 65–66
standard reviews
    See narrative reviews
standardised mean difference 101
study design 36
    See also randomised controlled trials (RCTs)
systematic reviews
    critique of 85–87, **86**
    data extraction in 43
    data synthesis in 43–45
    descriptive synthesis in 91
    dissemination of findings in 46–47, 129
    inclusion criteria in 38–40, 86
    overview 29–30, 32–33
    presentation and discussion of results in 45–46
    quality assessment in 41–43
    review protocol and 33–34
    review question, aim, and objective in 34–37
    study selection in 40–41, *41*
    types of literature reviews and 13
    writing and 5

textbooks 55
thematic analysis 15, 24, 90, 96–98, **97**
theoretical frameworks 75, 82
theoretical literature 52, 63
thesauruses 55
titles 74, 112
topic relevance 42–43
topics
    literature sources and 51–56, **54**
    selection of 48–51
traditional reviews
    See narrative reviews

UK Cochrane Centre (formerly Cochrane Centre in Oxford) 11

validity 76
Vancouver referencing system 126–127
veracity 77

writing
    overview 111–117
    quantitative research and 74
    systematic reviews and 5, 46